"Miriam Edelson's journey with her son Jake is a touching and vivid account of parenting under extraordinary circumstances. She prods, pushes, pulls and inspires movement with all systems in an effort to secure Jake's fragile future. In that regard, Edelson clearly emerges as an effective and intelligent advocate; a woman of significant faith; and an inspiration for parents. This book touches the heart, focuses the pain and highlights the challenge . . . a tribute to Jake that will last an eternity."

  – Bruce Rivers, Executive Director, Children's Aid Society
    of Toronto

"I deeply admire Miriam Edelson's ability to help us comprehend, in a breathtakingly honest account, the complexity and ambiguity of human lives and emotions. Much more than a memoir or a guide to families, the book contains a valid, and forceful, ethical argument for social commitment to the care of children with complex medical needs. Parents cannot be left alone to keep their children alive, nor to be abandoned. This book should be required reading for every policy-maker and health-care practitioner. Its insights will infuse our discussions and support for families."

  – Laura Shanner, Ph.D., University of Alberta,
    Health Ethics Centre

D1205225

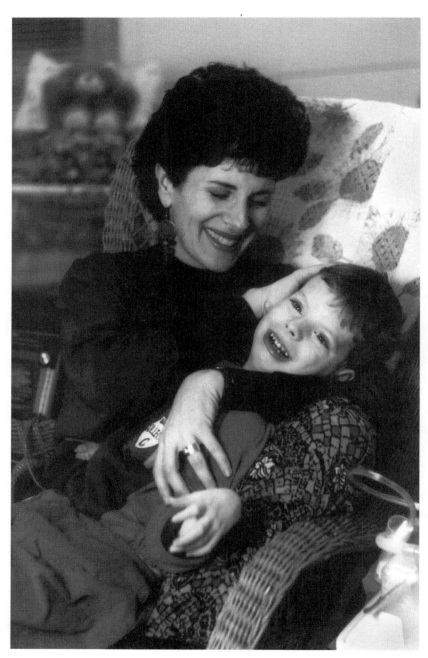

Jake at 5½ years old, with his mom at the group home.

MIRIAM EDELSON

My Journey with Jake

A Memoir of
Parenting and Disability

Between the Lines

My Journey with Jake

First published in Canada by
Between the Lines
720 Bathurst Street, Suite #404
Toronto, Ontario M5S 2R4
Second printing, March 2001

Canadian Cataloguing in Publication Data

Edelson, Miriam, 1956–
    My journey with Jake : a memoir of parenting and disability

ISBN 1-896357-35-0

1. Edelson, Jake – Health.   2. Edelson, Miriam, 1956–   .
3. Handicapped children – Care – Canada.
4. Handicapped children – Canada – Biography.
5. Parents of handicapped children – Canada – Biography.   I. Title.

HV890.C3E32 2000   362.4'092   C00-930235-2

Photo credits: courtesy of the author—pp. ii, 189; Jim Chorostecki—pp. 2, 27, 87, 92, 95, 99, 104, 114, 168; Mark Krakowski—pp. 79, 155; David Hartman—pp. 117, 144, 180, 185; Jay Chorostecki—p. 123

Text design by Gordon Robertson
Printed in Canada by union labour

Between the Lines gratefully acknowledges assistance for its publishing activities from the Canada Council for the Arts, the Ontario Arts Council, and the Government of Canada through the Book Publishing Industry Development Program.

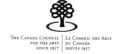

Dedicated with love to my daughter
Emma-Maryse Edelson Chorostecki

Behold, how good and how pleasant it is
when brothers and sisters dwell together in unity.

    — PSALM 133

Contents

Acknowledgements

J UST AS I AM FORTUNATE to live and work among a broad community of family, friends and colleagues, this book came to life thanks to the contributions of many individuals. June Callwood, Matt Cohen, Michael Enright, Katie FitzRandolph, Karen Levine, Malcolm Lester, Leo and Melanie Panitch, Laura Sky, Beverley Slopen, and Fern Valin read very early drafts and encouraged me to keep writing. Writer Rhea Tregebov provided valuable guidance early on.

My good friends Gary Cwitco, Andy King, Jane Finlay-Young, Gail Bench-Grant, Hinda Goldberg, Catharine Macleod, Morna McLeod, Frank Rooney, and Joy Woolfrey read later versions, offering many helpful comments and suggestions. The poet and short story writer Elisabeth Harvor worked patiently with me on the manuscript, through the auspices of the Humber School for Writers.

My wonderful midwives, Vicky Van Wagner and Elizabeth Allemang, helped me to decipher hospital records. Photographs by Jake's father, Jim Chorostecki, and by our dear friend Mark Krakowski, appear in these pages along with those taken by photographer David Hartman. I am grateful to each of them.

Gail Bench-Grant and the staff at Jake's group home, Susie's Place, continue to demonstrate an astounding depth of commitment to all the children in their care. It is the constancy of their support that allows me to tell Jake's story.

Jamie Swift, Ruth Bradley-St-Cyr, and Paul Eprile of Between the Lines brought this project to fruition. Thanks to my editors Trish O'Reilly and Julie Beddoes for helping to make the story far more compelling. My colleague John Ward contributed his finely-honed proofreading skills. I also gratefully acknowledge the Canada Council, the Ontario Arts Council, and the Roeher Institute for their support.

In addition, I must thank Paul Bilodeau and my colleagues at the Ontario Public Service Employees Union (as well as many other social justice activists across the country) who never hesitate to stop me and ask warmly, "How's Jake doing?" I am touched by the many expressions of genuine concern his story continues to evoke.

I want to thank Bob White, my friend and mentor, for teaching me never to back down from a worthwhile fight. My friend and union brother André Bekerman took precious time between cancer treatments to copy edit an early version of the manuscript. My appreciation to journalist Tom Walkom for believing in me and in the value of telling Jake's story.

I must also thank my friends, near and far—and you know who you are—who gathered round the birthing of this book, offering encouragement, insight and memories at the best and worst of moments in the process. Many a tear shared over the telephone line helped to keep me on track.

To Andy, I am grateful for thoughtful analysis (not to mention delicious home-cooked meals and occasional childcare) during this last year of intensive writing. His constancy and passion are truly a source of profound joy.

Finally I wish to thank my parents, Howard and Jacqueline Edelson, who are among the best editors I know, for their love and generosity. Any errors or omissions are, of course, my own.

1

Maiden Voyage

AN INTRAVENOUS FEEDING LINE is threaded through a plastic bubble perched on our newborn baby's head, the only site on his body where a large enough vein can be found. He is tiny and helpless. I am shocked by the multitude of tubes that, entwined round him like an exit ramp on a freeway, connect to various appliances. Some beep, others hum, their brightly coloured dials almost seeming to light a path by which our boy might wander out of this strange universe.

Groggy from an anaesthetic I meet our little son for the first time. Weighing less than six pounds, he is resting in a clear plastic rectangular box on wheels. It is the size of a small suitcase. The nurse assures me that he is snug as a bug but needs to be watched closely for respiratory distress.

Baby Jake is resting, the warmth of a pale blue knit cap offering him, I hope, some measure of comfort. He is fighting valiantly, making a difficult, meandering journey into our world. The nurses will not yet let me hold him—the danger of infection is too great. But, they say, I can start expressing breast milk to help sustain him. For the time being, he takes small amounts of water through the intravenous line. Burrowed in the transparent isolette, he resembles a

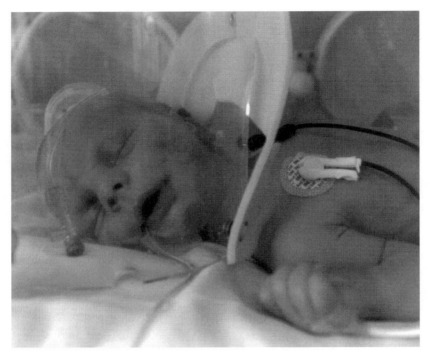

Jake, one day old.

creature descended from outer space—except that because of the unexpected Caesarean birth, his head is perfectly shaped.

My baby's abrupt separation from my body is a jarring break from the nine months I carried him securely in my belly. If I were not so in need of healing time myself, I suspect I would feel even more at a loose end. We are able to stroke him gently through small, antiseptic apertures that open like portholes on the side of his spaceship. He does not flinch from our touch. Still, the absence of the baby in my arms, at my breast, thwarts a most primal urge. At certain moments, I experience an overwhelming desire to spirit him away from this terrible place.

I have been awakened soon after leaving post-op because two-hours-old Jake is to be transported to the neonatal intensive care unit at the Hospital for Sick Children next door. An obstetrics nurse will guide his gurney through the tunnels, accompanied by my husband Jim, his hand placed protectively over his son's torso, nearly covering the body, smaller than a football.

The next morning, I make my first visit to Sick Kids, where Jake lies wired up in his clear plastic box. Jim pushes me in the wheelchair after the nurse has hauled me out of bed to lumber the short distance to the washroom. On the maternity ward in Toronto General, rooms are overflowing with mothers, their babies, breasts and families. The atmosphere is joyful, teeming with life and hope.

It feels a bit strange to sit in a rocking chair amid all the equipment in the neonatal intensive care unit. Jake reclines across a pillow on my knees like a jewel on a cushion. The nurses try to make me feel comfortable but I feel clumsy, an inexperienced new mother trying to nurse, on display. Our maple rocking chair, so carefully chosen a few short weeks ago, sits idle in the nursery at home.

We are too concerned about Jake's health to waste much energy on regrets. Jake emerged blue from my belly, his lungs and throat full of mucus. Able hands quickly transferred him to a workstation about a dozen steps away. A team of three professionals tried to kick-start his breathing by inserting a tube down through his nose into his lungs to suction out mucus. They gave him an oxygen mask because he was not breathing spontaneously, his lungs evidently quite wet. Some resuscitation was required and, at thirty minutes old, a tube was inserted down into the trachea to deliver oxygen right into his lungs to guard them from collapse.

Apparently many babies born by Caesarean section require suctioning as fluid is not squeezed from the lungs by the journey through the birth canal. Jake's breathing difficulties alone were not cause for spectacular alarm. Apgar scores, based on tests performed on all newborns, were okay. They measured his colour, heart rate, reflex response and muscle tone. After half an hour of intense work by highly specialized physicians, Jake's chest was clear and his heart sounded normal. His blood gases measurement reflected reasonable health and he displayed the sucking reflex. It was noted that he arched his back, tossing his head and eyes upwards but it is his problem with breathing that leads to his transfer to intensive care at Sick Kids.

When Jake is two days old, I am allowed to nurse him a few times a day. Three or four days after his birth, however, we still have no idea how long it will be before we can all go home. We assume this is a momentary glitch. Our families and close friends come to my room in Toronto General and express love and concern; we tell them what we know. Some also visit the neonatal unit at Sick Kids to take a peek but only members of the immediate family may don sterile gowns and enter the inner sanctum of care.

Meanwhile, my hospital room bustles with activity. I am earnestly expressing breast milk, with the help of a nurse who takes a shine to us once she learns that both Jim and I are union people. She ensures that I know how to wield the industrial-sized electric pump properly and stops in regularly to chat. I am reassured by the experience she shares so generously.

It is spring. My father-in-law from Sarnia has sent a pot of blue hydrangeas that spruce up the room beautifully. As always, buds on the trees usher in hope for a good year, for new beginnings. I am feeling well, gradually more mobile after the first couple of Demerol-drip days following surgery.

The cause of Jake's condition is still not known. I am excited about his birth and our new life together as a family. I wonder, as I pump milk from my breast into a sterile plastic bottle, whether this separation from him will affect the bonding process I have read so much about. Jim walks the precious bottles over to our boy at Sick Kids a few times a day. We have to trust that Nature is sufficiently wise to adapt to such unusual situations. I do so miss my baby's soothing presence inside me.

I gave birth to my beautiful strawberry blond, blue-eyed boy on April 18, 1990. It was a time of great optimism in my life. I was thirty-four and life had already thrown me a couple of curves but I genuinely believed that Jim, my partner, and I had turned a significant corner. In my mind at least, raising this child together represented our faith in a delicious future. The pregnancy was unremarkable. I was a fit, healthy woman with no discernible physical difficulties. My spirits were buoyant. At the predestined time, music played in the softly lit hospital birthing room. Two labour coaches, as well as our doctor, accompanied Jim and me. "Breathe me Vicky,"

I remember panting emphatically, imploring our midwife to remain close, to lock her eyes with mine while the strongest contractions rocked my body. After twenty-six hours I was longing to bear down and push out my long-awaited child.

Then, the hospital's chief obstetrician arrived. After a cursory greeting, he plunged a gloved hand in to examine my gaping cervix. It hurt like hell. I responded with language that was, no doubt, unbecoming of a lady. The two medical men had a quiet word in the corner and then our own doctor told us firmly, but with great compassion, that the baby was stuck, unable to turn its head. Jake was presenting face first, a rare incidence. This was problematic since normally the baby tucks its head forward, presenting the smallest area possible which allows it to slide more easily down the birth canal. With Jake's head flexed back, no amount of pushing would allow him to emerge safely. Even our midwife agreed that an emergency C- section was required.

In seconds, the birth was transformed. Jim and I were swept from the relative calm of the birthing room into a stainless steel operating theatre. I remember feeling cheated at not being able to experience the culminating moments of pushing, that coveted prize promised to women who successfully endure hour upon hour of unrelenting contractions.

There was no time to dwell on this thought, however; my birth canal had become an unsafe place. I was prodded and poked, given a heavy-duty shot of Demerol between contractions so the surgeon could slice through seven layers of muscle and retrieve the baby.

Jake's first days in hospital were intense. Doctors and nurses poked more needles through his tiny feet and head than the average tattoo parlour artist. More plastic tubing was stuffed up his nose in seven days than most of us experience in a lifetime. And he lost more than a pound during those first few days, a greater fluctuation than normally expected.

I now understand that the medical emergency at Jake's birth was also a defining moment for me as a parent. I experienced early what comes to every parent: the release of control that our children demand of us as they grow. There is, in fact, no grand plan. We give them life, but raise them in conditions not entirely of our making.

In another era, Jake most certainly would have died at birth or soon after. Only my womb's complex ecosystem was fashioned so that he might flourish. Inside me, he was well. The outside world cannot sustain him.

Seven days have passed and Jake is ready to leave the Hospital for Sick Children. He is now off the respirator though his breathing is laboured. While he is still connected to an intravenous line for hydration and antibiotics, he is digesting tiny amounts of breast milk. The jaundice he experienced soon after birth is dissipating. He can now be cared for at a less acute neonatal unit. He is being transferred to St. Joseph's Health Centre, about a forty-minute walk from our home.

That evening at home I can soak in a luxurious hot bath now that the staples are removed from my belly. Afterward, I am resting quietly while Jim puts away groceries in the kitchen. It feels like we're just beginning to resume the normal rhythm of our lives—except, of course, that Jake is not yet strong enough to come home. When the phone rings, I can tell by the flatness of Jim's voice that the call is from the hospital.

He enters the bedroom, shaken. He sits down next to me on our bed, searching for the right words. It seems that just before leaving The Hospital for Sick Children, Jake had, for some reason, been given a CT scan. The results are not good. There are marks indicating calcifications on the brain, and the *corpus callosum*, a key brain component, is missing entirely.

All sense of relief at being home suddenly evaporates. We are silent for a moment then hold one another and cry. Mustering our courage, we make our way to St. Joe's where our newborn son is being taken by ambulance. We are told, by neurologist Dr. Mehta, that Jake is scheduled for frequent neurological exams to chart his development; he will have tests to check for seizure activity in his brain. Doctors will check to see if he is reaching major milestones at the usual times. Is he starting to hold up his head? Does he track the movement when a finger is waved before his eyes? We will see Dr. Mehta again when Jake is fourteen weeks old.

For the next three days I will spend part of each day at St. Joe's but at home I move into action mode. I make many phone calls to search out answers to our endless questions. No one knows exactly what the CT scan results will mean for Jake's future—certainly learning disabilities and perhaps seizures. Only time will tell. I get us on the epilepsy association mailing list, sign Jake up for physiotherapy and a special needs nursery program. Meanwhile, beyond our own crisis spot in the world, the sun continues to rise and set.

I nurse Jake several times a day at the hospital and express breast milk at home. Attached to the big breast pump we rent, I muse at my new role as milch cow. I gradually begin to feel joyful at the possibility of ordinary mothering.

Sometimes I walk near the hospital between feedings. The streets are crowded with outdoor markets, flowers, and strolling residents enjoying the spring. Our community includes many Eastern European immigrants and young families. Jim and I felt comfortable settling here, with our own roots in Poland and Eastern Europe connecting us somehow to our neighbours in the pungent delicatessens and pastry shops that line the main streets.

I stop for coffee and skim my newspaper. I imagine that soon Jake and I will spend hours like this together, wandering around the park, exploring the boutiques as I did before he was born. A straw basket with fresh white linen and mini-mattress stands ready by our bed. The change table is poised to receive our little man at a moment's notice; a black and white mobile my nieces have outgrown dangles above. The cloth diaper service is on standby. Jake's baby pouch hangs ready on a hook by the door. We are ready for anything, I think.

After ten hard days in two neonatal facilities, Jake is finally strong enough to come home. His breathing is still laboured but he is beginning to open his eyes for more than a few minutes at a time and to look around, as if sagely. Without all the plastic tubes and bubbles attached to his head from the neonatal ICU, he looks like a beautiful perfect baby. When I place the woven rainbow cap on his head, my earlier image of Jake from outer space dissipates for good. As we trundle out of the hospital, encumbered with all that matters to us in the world, my spirits are strong.

The very first evening at home has a warm spring feel. We wrap Jake up in a colourful receiving blanket, his arms pressed close to his sides, the way that infants most like. Only his perfect head, topped with the multi-coloured cotton knit cap, is showing. We walk to a folk concert at a nearby church. People stop to admire him and chat. Jake's skin tastes sweet, his baby smell so alluring. Surrounded by music, he hardly makes a peep. His arduous maiden voyage into our world has finally achieved lift-off.

2

Hard-wired for kids

I CANNOT REMEMBER A TIME that I didn't expect to have children of my own. I genuinely enjoy kids, particularly toddlers. In university, I occasionally purchased children's books that I found appealing. I remember admiring *Show Me*, a somewhat controversial European book about sexuality for children. It cost me more than I contributed weekly to the grocery kitty in our co-op house. Twenty-three years later my daughter Emma and I finally cracked the cover to spend an evening leafing through it together.

It's as if I was hard-wired for kids.

In my family, it was expected that we youngsters would one day have children of our own. It's what people did. Bringing children into the world, to build a better tomorrow, was a *mitzvah*—a cause for celebration.

Just as strongly, my parents insisted that we should "make a contribution," no matter what we decided to do in the world. This credo ran deep. Whether in science, medicine, journalism or teaching, one would contribute to making the world a better place. I remember many a dinner table conversation about people who were making a difference: Rosa Parks and Martin Luther King in the civil rights movement; the four students gunned down at Kent State;

Lester Pearson and the Canadian peacekeeping forces. The spirit of these people and the ideals they espoused were present in our home in a suburb outside New York City.

In 1968, my mother placed a bronze-coloured sculpture on the piano in our living room. It depicted a Vietnamese woman holding her baby and a gun, standing in a field. A look of defiance was etched on her face. Soon after, my parents decided to leave New York and settle in Toronto where my mother's family lived. She had been raised in Canada and they hoped to build a better life for us, away from the violence of American society. I was twelve and this meant less to me than leaving my beloved New York Mets behind. (Their fortunes were stalled in the cellar until the year after we moved to Canada when they won the World Series—my only regret at having moved.) Notwithstanding these youthful preoccupations, the notion of social responsibility remained firmly ingrained when the time came to venture out on my own. My parents had laid a solid, secular basis on which to discern right from wrong.

A cartoon from the *New Yorker* magazine was displayed prominently in the kitchen of the house my parents bought in Toronto in the summer of 1968. It pictured a man sitting on the ledge of a tall building. His wife is looking out the window imploring him, "It's all right. We'll move to Canada so you won't have to choose between Humphrey and Nixon." Humour was a welcome guest in our household and the cartoon reflected my parents' sensibilities. They were engaged by politics and social issues, if not always actively, then certainly in lively discussion around the dinner table.

Nonetheless, the message about creating family remained very strong. Although it was never expected I would go to university just to meet a husband, if that had happened, I doubt anyone would have complained. While I lived in Ottawa during the eighties, working full-time in the trade union movement and completing my master's thesis during holidays, my parents were always interested in discussing union issues. But now that my career was moving, they wanted me to get married and have children.

Today, I understand this desire for little people much better, but back then the pressure could have been a good deal more subtle. As I approached thirty I began dreading that part of the visit home when I could expect the third degree. On one trip, I arrived in Toronto with a special gift for my parents. It was a red-haired, blue-eyed Cabbage Patch doll. I told them her name was Sarah Rachel and that she would be their Cabbage Patch grandchild. After that, they stayed off my back for some time. When I did have my own kids, Sarah Rachel was pressed into active service, as a playmate for little ones visiting Grandma and Grampa's house.

The notion of making a contribution was my mother's way of saying that her daughter would do both career and family, just as she had. She often told me that she had already fought feminist battles. In the forties she convinced her own rather conservative father to allow her to attend graduate school in social work in the United States. She was subsequently active in early union organizing among social workers, advocating collective, rather than individually-based, solutions to societal problems.

My father worked mainly in sales of arts and crafts materials for schools and camps. He is an avid reader and primarily self-educated. Literature, economics, and history are his strong suits. He always stressed to us that going to university was a privilege not to be missed.

As a university student living in another city, I often brought home my essays for my father to read. I would wait while he read and commented on the hypotheses I advanced in my philosophy or history papers. Even in high school, my brothers and I had often talked through ideas for term papers with one or both of my parents. We did the research and writing ourselves, but the discussion with them encouraged us to think critically and to question authority. I know I always struggled to produce something worthy of my father's praise. My parents taught us that we could change the world if we applied ourselves and worked collectively.

I was proud to work for the Public Service Alliance of Canada (PSAC), the union that represents federal public service workers. I never believed we were making the revolution, but I certainly felt we were working on the side of justice. My job involved being part of a team of organizers on Parliament Hill, teaching education programs and assisting members and union locals to solve problems in their workplaces.

My primary interest was developing the union's women's program. I helped organize a series of educational conferences across the country. We also worked to put in place internal affirmative action programs aimed at increasing women's involvement at all levels to make the union a more inclusive organization. I wrote several articles about the barriers to women's participation in unions; some of these were used by PSAC and the Canadian Union of Public Employees (CUPE) in member education programs. As it always had, writing offered me a chance to step back and reflect, to try and make sense of my experiences in life and on the job.

In the early eighties, I fell in love with a charming Franco-Ontarian activist and Alliance member. His daughter, Manon, was eleven when her father and I became involved. Over the next couple of years, I found her exuberance absolutely delightful and became very attached to her. When I realised my lover did not want another child, I felt devastated. It's likely our relationship lasted as long as it did because I could not bear losing Manon from my life.

When her father and I finally did part, keeping contact with her proved complicated. It was not something he encouraged. She was also starting high school and had a full slate of activities. I felt that I had no choice but to back off, despite my sense of loss.

After this heartbreak, I lived in a third floor flat in a house owned by friends from graduate school. Like many in our circle, much of my social life was centred on labour council activities, protests and political debate. But I was twenty-seven and the noisy ticking of my biological clock was a constant distraction. I had a good job and some close friends but I wondered when I would meet a life partner.

Jim and I first met in spring 1983 at a staff conference for the Alliance. Over three days cooped up in a conference plenary room with our colleagues, we passed notes and laughed in fits and starts. He liked my wry wit. I enjoyed his sunny personality. A certain irreverence fuelled our easy banter and we became friends. I worked in Hull, he was based in Toronto, and we did similar jobs for the union; education, organizing, and dealing with member grievances kept us extremely busy.

The unrelenting pace of labour movement activity takes its toll on one's health. Not long after a successful year-long organizing campaign at the Library of Parliament in 1984, the year in which I also completed my MA thesis, I experienced my first bout of burnout. Not realizing then how quickly exhaustion can spiral into dark debilitating depression, I ignored the warning signs for some time. To stave off worry and insomnia, I increased my exercise routine. I ate well and didn't drink much, but weight began to fall off my body. I felt anxious all the time and had moments where I felt disoriented. I was often tearful, but didn't recognize this as a symptom. Once, after several days of fitful sleep, I fainted during a meeting. Finally, I went to see my doctor. She said that I needed to retreat from the day-to-day pressures of the job, believing I was cruising for a serious breakdown.

My favourite retreat from the pace of work was to spend time beside a serene lake in the Gatineau Hills, just one hour from town. In 1981, a group of my friends had put our savings together and bought this property. We called it, simply, the land. Luckily, I was able to spend several weeks there, gradually replenishing my resources. I was able to re-establish my inner sense of equilibrium. The natural beauty helped me feel well, as it would many times in the years to come.

When Jim moved to Ottawa in 1985, we began to work out, skate and cross-country ski together. Gradually, we were becoming soul mates, although we remained only friends. I felt safe with him, in part because I never expected anything more than companionship.

Later that year, after his relationship broke up, we began to see one another romantically. Our friends and colleagues were surprised. Some were upset that Jim and his former partner had separated. We were able to get away from the gossip at the lake in summer 1986, chopping wood and hauling water for cooking. (I felt this to be a quintessential Canadian activity.) It was clear that Jim knew how to relax. I did not, but I was desperately trying to learn. Taking it easy was not something we learned in my family. Achievement and accomplishments were valued above all, as in many ethnic groups that have emigrated to North America or lived through the hardships of the thirties.

At the land, I carried pails of lake water up a steep slope to our campsite. Maintaining the woodpile had always been my job. Jim helped drag fallen logs from the bush so that I could split them. We slept in a tent and cooked over the open wood fire. Hours were spent sunning in the nude on a huge rock that overhangs the water, with no one in sight but waterfowl and the occasional curious squirrel. We managed to slow down to a pace that mirrored the day's rhythm.

This was definitely my territory. This secluded spot in the woods bred magic for me and the surroundings helped to nurture an easy intimacy between Jim and me. We watched shooting stars at night and scanned the lake for birds through a telescope during the early morning mist. Driving into town for supplies at dusk, we honed eagle eyes on the bush surrounding us, occasionally sighting deer scampering just off the dusty, dirt road.

Jim's sunny disposition and firm grasp of life's practical aspects provided a good complement to my own nature. I had become aware of my location on the margins, particularly in Ottawa, as a rather intense, left-wing Jewish woman. I liked how it felt to fit in, something Jim did so easily. The sense that we made a good team was growing in meaning for both of us.

Soon after Jim and I began to see one other, his mother died suddenly. I happened to be in Saskatoon for a PSAC women's conference. Jim contacted me at a mutual colleague's where we were finishing supper and discussing the next day's workshops.

"My mother died last night," Jim said. "I need you to be with me."

"I'll get the next flight out," I said, without hesitation.

Later, at Jim's family home in Sarnia, Ontario, the first time I met any of his family, his father John, his brothers and their wives sorted out the funeral plans, a somber evening.

Watching him interact with his family, I was struck by Jim's integrity. He is the eldest son. As we sat around the dinner table, each person speaking what was in his heart, Jim acted as facilitator, making sure that each person's views were listened to with both warmth and decorum.

The service was held next day at the church where John and his wife had worshipped and sung in the choir. The whole family was there. No one was prepared for this untimely death, especially cruel since John was soon to retire, hoping to spend more time with his wife, exploring Lake Huron from the deck of their brand new sailboat cruiser. It was not meant to be.

One of Jim's brothers began to read a passage of scripture; when he started to cry, he passed the book over to his wife who, without skipping a beat, finished the reading. I was moved by the evident strength of the connection between them. The children sang and spoke of their grandmother. Afterwards, we returned to the family home with the relatives and close friends for refreshments and remembrances. It was very quiet.

A year or so after we became lovers, Jim's promotion led to a move to Toronto. Although moving so far from the land was at first unthinkable for me, it seemed a good career move for us both. The initial thought was that we would only stay for two years and then return to Ottawa. It seemed wise for me to work for a different union and I found work as Executive Director of the CBC National Radio Producers Association (NRPA), which represented journalists across the country, outside Quebec.

We had a blast, enjoying the busy cultural activities in the big city. We joined the Y, minutes from my downtown workplace. It was a comfortable time in our relationship, with few responsibilities other than work and an exciting city to explore. We decided to get married, excited by the prospect of raising a family. We were married on February 12, 1988, in the home we were house sitting for our friend Mark. It was a simple and secular ceremony, followed by a banquet given by my parents. We also planned a simpler get together at our home. Through a friend, I asked if the Fly By Night Dyke Band would play at our wedding party, but they declined, apparently for ideological reasons!

At the more traditional wedding banquet, Jim's father introduced a Polish wedding song and to his great surprise (and ours) a contingent of my mother's friends and colleagues joined in the Polish singing. Many of the women were Holocaust survivors; this astonishing linkage of cultures—across barriers historical and lived—was a sheer delight.

At work I was helping to negotiate some of the early job-sharing contracts at the CBC. These allowed women to continue in their demanding positions without losing seniority or benefits, while working fewer hours each week. From time to time, I run into former members and it's great when they thank me for helping them achieve a reasonable balance between their professional and family responsibilities. It was a time of great learning and very gratifying personally and professionally.

A short time after our marriage, Jim and I bought part of a duplex jointly with my brother and his family. This brought me close to our young nieces. Before her second birthday, Kaitlyn often climbed the stairs to our apartment looking for her Aunt Mir. She was two when her parents had to head to the hospital for the birth of a new baby. In our living room little Kate was dancing with us all, around and around in a circle, to bright music playing on the stereo. Her parents gradually moved closer to the door and left unobtrusively. Sister Sarah arrived while Kate was sound asleep in her bed, seemingly unperturbed by her parents' furtive departure.

In later months, Jim often walked Sarah patiently around our home, trying to help her settle while her parents were out for an evening. Jim is a big man, but a very gentle soul. Babies love to be in his arms, drawn in close to the warmth of his body. Definitely a natural safe harbour.

Very early in our friendship, before we became lovers, Jim and I had talked about wanting children. For him, it was a fairly recent desire. As I was approaching thirty (which then seemed incredibly old), and because of my earlier experience with Manon's father,

Jim's interest in starting a family one day was important to me. My painful parting with Manon meant that the knowledge of losing a child was present in my psyche when my niece Kaitlyn and her family moved away from the duplex we shared. Spending time with her, I had become aware how much I wanted to be a mother to a child who would stay with me always. It was soon after my brother's family moved that Jim and I decided it was time to start our own.

During my pregnancy with Jake, I thought a lot about the children I had loved earlier in my life, before I felt ready to have one of my own. As I swam or cross-country skied with Jim, I finally felt like the woman I'd always wanted to be: strong, fit and wonderfully grounded. Burnout and depression were ancient history. I was a woman with a sharp focus and a bright future ahead. We anticipated nothing but good health in days to come.

3

Searching for Answers

B Y THE TIME Jake is almost five weeks old at the end of May we appear to be healing from our respective traumas. My scar no longer resembles the Grand Canyon and Jake seems to be feeding better. The beginnings of a natural care pharmacy are overtaking the bathroom counter where the vitamin E oil for my belly joins the calendula cream destined both to soothe nursing nipples and clean Jake's scalp.

Jim is back at work; Jake and I spend our days at home, with frequent walks to catch some mild spring air. In between feeding and changing Jake, there is not much time. Jim, who has done housework from a young age, races home most evenings to be with his son.

My days are also crowded with Jake's medical appointments at St. Joe's. As well, once a week we cross the city for cranio-sacral massage therapy treatments to relieve muscle and nerve trauma caused by the abnormal position of Jake's neck during birth. The therapist is caring for his own newborn baby on days when he isn't in the office. His scientific approach is infused with warmth for the client. After all the hospital waiting rooms we have come to know intimately during recent weeks, the humanity of this complementary health care practitioner is truly comforting.

I sit near my son as the therapist sets him down carefully on a deep blue, cushion-top table. Jake seems to enjoy the gentle touch. He sleeps or coos sweetly as skilled hands work on his tiny, malleable body. But the muscle tone in Jake's neck is terribly weak. It is too soon to know if he is "developmentally delayed," one of the new terms I've learned.

We speak quietly of our new family members, comparing notes on their sleep patterns and nursing routines. Afterwards I walk long distances, drinking in the spring air. I am still hesitant to drive much with him and take the subway, his head nestled against my chest. The motion puts him to sleep and I enjoy the walk back home through the quiet streets near the park.

My scar is healing but my energy, like that of all new mothers, is low. Fortunately, I've been able to swim occasionally since three weeks after surgery; it helps me keep up with the extra stress of Jake's feeding and myriad of appointments. We never settle into much of a routine. At seven or eight weeks, he still hasn't cracked a smile, even though the baby care books promise this reward for taking such good care of our baby. I wonder if my fatigue stems from the waning of pure adrenaline that carried us through those first ten days in hospital.

For the first time since leaving my parents' home at age eighteen, I have little control over my schedule. I feel I've managed to accomplish a few things out there in the world and this exhausted, rather bovine existence, is completely alien. I feel rather unstrung and doubt I'm capable of nurturing even a rhododendron. Jake's feeding problems, which merit a chapter to themselves, add greatly to my anxiety and sense of failure at not having produced a perfect child.

I fear I am again sliding into a depression. I know the effect prolonged sleep interruption has on my body and psyche. I am a bundle of nerves, my body veering out of my control. I am fortunate to have women in my support network who tell me what every mother needs to know—that I'm not alone in feeling how I do. But the gruelling round of hospital and clinic appointments and all my unanswered questions about Jake's condition, make this more than the usual new mother's stress.

I am frequently tearful. My thoughts race madly. I feel as if I couldn't string together a coherent sentence if my life depended on it. Sleep is elusive and fitful. I can laugh with Jim, somewhat wryly, that I am sleep-*depraved*, but we both know these signals are not to be ignored.

Our family physician recognizes the pre-burnout warning signs. Even without a very sick infant, the interrupted sleep pattern could spirit me into a dark, downward spiral. She thinks we can stop this, for Jake's benefit and my own. She asks if I am still swimming, knowing how much the release of physical energy helps me to handle stress. This is different than the usual postpartum depression. She recommends we apply for minor assistance through the public home care system.

To get home care, your doctor must register you with an agency and a file is only activated once you become a "case" in the system. This means that you need help to care for your child and must answer personal questions about everything from family income to laundry habits. For obvious reasons this can be rather humbling. We mothers are supposed to be able to handle it all. (Unless you are independently wealthy, in which case you can just hire the help without the evaluation.) Nonetheless, for Jake and for me, it is more prudent to swallow my pride.

The next step, about two weeks later, is an evaluation by the home care agency. One afternoon after I've scoured the bathroom and kitchen between feedings and sessions with the breast pump, a social worker comes to the house to make an assessment of our needs. Her demeanour is professional, somewhat distant. She knows that Jake is likely to have neurological problems as he grows. I hold him in my arms as we sit in the living room. I am determined to make a good impression.

"I take it your husband is at work during the day," she says.

"Oh yes," I say, trying to evoke June Cleaver in my responses. I don't mention that Ward—that is, Jim—also frequently works evenings.

"And does little Jake sleep through the night yet?"

"Not usually," I answer, trying not to sound too concerned. Of course, I'm wondering whether we get more points or less for a ten-week-old who only sleeps a few hours at a time.

"Hmm," she pauses, writing something in her notebook.

"Does he startle?" she asks.

"Pardon me?" I say. What is this woman on about, I wonder? Suddenly she claps her hands loudly near Jake's head.

He literally rises to the occasion and stirs. Now I *am* curious. Is this a good thing, or some ghastly new deficit she's discovered?

After a few more questions, she says, "All right, Mrs. Edelson. That's all for now. I'll make my report and you'll hear from the agency in a week or two."

"Thank you," I say, showing her to the door. The only *Mrs.* Edelson I know is my mother.

A health care aide is assigned to us two afternoons a week and I am free to leave the house unaccompanied. I admit—not proudly—that I feel like a jailbird released on parole.

It is painfully clear that we are able to benefit from this publicly funded service only because our family doctor knew how to intervene on our behalf. She and I both caught the signs of risk to my own physical and mental health in time. Jim and I could not afford to pay for such help without assistance. I suspect that many new mothers under similar stress do not get the help they need.

The health care aides who arrive at our door at one o'clock on Tuesday and Thursday afternoons are almost all recent immigrants. Some are nurses or midwives in their countries of origin—the Philippines, Jamaica or Guatemala—but their qualifications are not recognized here. They work a four-hour shift and do a couple of loads of laundry, as well as watch Jake.

The first day, I greet the woman at the door and then show her Jake's bedroom and the laundry room. She asks a couple of questions while meeting the baby and hearing about our household routines. During the first two weeks of this new regime, a different woman arrives for each shift. So much turnover is disconcerting given Jake's special challenges and need (his and mine) for continuity. It also means that my anxiety level is not completely relieved as I leave him with another stranger. Just because you have cabin fever doesn't mean you can leave the cabin easily.

But still, twice a week I can head down to the Y for a soothing swim. Afterwards, I do errands downtown or meet a friend for coffee. I am trying to keep some contact with the rest of the world but it's hard when Jake needs such constant attention. Complete isolation is not good for anybody. Although it takes an effort to step out of the strange, medically-driven time capsule that I've been living in, I force myself.

Other days, I take Jake with me to the Y. We drive down together on the heels of the frenetic Toronto rush hour and I leave him upstairs for an hour in the babysitting service. The women are very friendly and get used to me calling them halfway through my work-out. He sleeps peacefully in the cribs they provide or, if he doesn't settle, they give him a bottle I've prepared. It takes me about an hour to blast the anxiety out of my body. No question, exercise and regular breaks help my mood and sleep.

After several weeks, I begin to feel like I'm more on top of things. Getting regular exercise and scheduled short breaks away from the house does wonders. I'm also enjoying the time at home with Jake more. One of the women assigned to us is coming regularly. Lilly and I begin to develop a rapport after she has cared for Jake a few times. She is a lovely Filipino-Canadian woman with a background in midwifery. She seems to connect with him.

One afternoon when I get home, Lilly tells me, "I'm sorry . . . I have a new job. As a nanny."

I am bowled over. Why would she choose to work as a nanny, with her qualifications? I am touched by her honesty. She didn't have to tell me. But I am also troubled that our public home care system is losing a skilled worker due, it seems, to inefficient scheduling and low wages. Moreover, now I must brace myself for yet another parade of health care aides into our home.

Jake has high needs and more than babysitting is required. My dad volunteers to watch his grandson while I do groceries or go for a jog through the park. I appreciate the gesture and we give it a try.

Jake sleeps a while in his grandfather's arms, but gets a bit cranky after that. I'm gone for less than an hour but it's too much for a seventy-three-year-old man. It has been a long time since my father cared for an infant, much less one not in top-notch condition.

My mother, several years younger and of a different temperament, is more able to anticipate an infant's needs but she is still employed full-time and cannot be on call for us. I suspect many new mothers find themselves in similar straits, without a lot of practical support on hand. You are stuck until you can build up some trades with friends or other families. This is hardly the carefree maternity leave I imagined. I have seven months off work and wonder what our lives will look like at the end of this phase. Our budget will not permit me to take more time off.

Much of my day—besides caring for my son—is still spent on the telephone; I call agencies such as the Epilepsy Foundation and the Association for Community Living to learn about services for children with special needs. I have virtually no experience with babies and little first-hand knowledge of disability. I also visit several child-care centres to check out their integrated programs and fill out a multitude of forms. We are now on several different waiting lists—ready, I think, for every conceivable eventuality.

The home care evaluation also recommended that Jake receive physiotherapy as an early intervention tool. There is a four-month waiting list. I am stunned. Everything I've read and learned from contacting self-help and support organizations suggests that the early months are most crucial to the infant's future capacity for development. Again I hit the phone lines, trying to find a way to short-circuit the waiting list. "Four months is not good enough," I tell anyone who will listen. "My son needs help now."

Jake's godmother Hinda puts us in touch with an occupational therapist who comes to the house and assesses Jake informally. She explains that he will need help learning to hold up his head. She gives us a program of exercises to do with him, stretching and strengthening movements to spur his development. She emphasizes that progress during these early months will be absolutely key to his future development.

We learn to roll Jake on a bright plastic beach ball, encouraging him to hold up his head. I crouch down, then lay him face down on the striped ball. We are just an arm's-length apart. When I roll the ball back toward my body, Jake lifts his head to look at me. He holds it for a moment, filling me with the hope that he can progress.

She also gives us information about feeding techniques for babies with swallowing and digestive difficulties. I wonder why we never saw these materials at the hospital or doctor's office. I can't help but wonder about the other babies on the physiotherapy waiting list. Not to make help widely available at the optimal time, in a country so rich with resources, seems criminal.

This is our first foray into what I soon recognize as "the mothering underground."

Another of Hinda's contacts is a woman who works as an early childhood education teacher at an integrated nursery school. She drops by one afternoon and we sit on the living room floor, Jake lying on a soft green receiving blanket draped over the rug. She shows me some carrying positions and movements that might also help Jake's muscles develop. She explains how parents can learn to move their own bodies, acting as "developmental furniture" for their special needs kids. Our sitting in a certain way will give Jake physical support but also challenge him to use his limbs.

She also describes a few creative sensory stimulation exercises for infants. I find this very encouraging. I sign us up for a playgroup at her nursery program, to begin in September. In the meantime, I scavenge fabric stores for swatches of material—from flannel to corduroy and silks, in different colours. At home or out in the park, I stroke Jake's hands and legs and face with the different fabrics, allowing him to experience a range of textures on his skin.

My friends Hinda and Jane are clearly the movers and shakers behind the mothering underground that brings these skilled women to our doorstep. Without them, I would be lost. They are devoted mothers to their own children and always make an extra effort to help out friends going through tough times. I am grateful to learn, through them, that there are resources out there in the community.

No one seems horrified by Jake or expresses pity for us. I feel uncertain and a bit afraid, but I learn, in part by example of the other mothers I meet, that we can deal with most challenges and help Jake face them too as he grows up.

Of course, a few people we know drop out of sight, perhaps distressed by Jake's apparent limits and the extent to which he consumes our attention. I realize later that not everyone has the interest or patience to deal with people whose lives are more tumultuous than usual.

I wonder how other mothers of special needs babies cope with these challenges, especially if they have other small children to care for. They must be seriously exhausted. Where do they get the time to research what care is available? What if they don't speak English well? It must be confusing—even terrifying—to have to find and use all these services. Even for me, it is tough in spite of the fact that I've honed my advocacy skills during twenty years of activism in the women's, student and trade union movements.

When Jake is about ten weeks old, Jim and I take him to Ottawa to meet our friends who make a big fuss over our little boy. On the weekend, we pack him up for a short jaunt to Montreal. The jazz festival is in full swing and we enjoy walking about, listening to music out of doors, with him in the Snugli. We even bundle him up one evening and brave a live concert of tango music. Jake behaves very well, much to the relief of our neighbours, and seems to enjoy the irresistible beat of Latin music.

Jim leaves on a business trip directly from Montreal while Jake and I embark upon an adventure of our own—the train. We board and find a couple of seats together where I can spread out our belongings. Jake is very quiet. He nurses a bit, and later I give him a bottle before he falls asleep. He seems quite content, relaxing to the rhythm of the train's gentle motion. I spend these few hours examining every crevice of my son's body. Like a mother cat, I practically lick my boy clean, observing his changes. We make it home in one piece, ready for a stretch on our own.

By the time Jake is almost four months old, I am again worn out. We have another set of tests coming up at St. Joe's and Jim isn't even

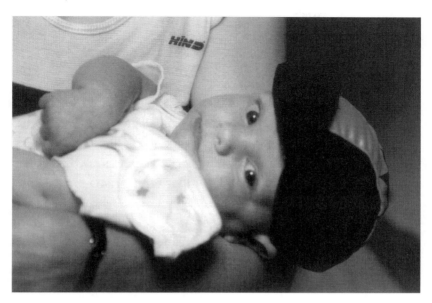

Jake the athlete, 4 months old.

going to be here. I feel like I'm carrying this all by myself. I still don't know what the CT scan results mean or what all these tests will tell us. Not knowing, of course, means I fear the worst. I can't sleep when the baby goes down and I'm running on empty. Sometimes, I'm just plain cranky. There is a part of me, my intellectual side, not fulfilled so far by this project. I'm not bucking to go out and negotiate a peace treaty between Israel and the Palestinians but, frankly, domestic bliss among the diaper pails is eluding me.

When Jim gets home, he is exhausted. He's pretty good about taking care of Jake during the evening, but I feel like he's shut down on me. He doesn't feel much like talking. I sure hope it's just a stage.

The winter before Jake's birth, we were all first-timers in the pre-natal group run by the midwives' collective. An easy rapport had developed in our class, all manner of questions asked and answered. One warm evening, we are gathering at one couple's home near the lake. As we enter, we are drawn right in to the festivities. We sit around the living room showing off our babies in their funny new hats. The talk is light, a reminder of the camaraderie developed during our eight Thursday evenings together. Everyone seems so relaxed in their new roles. Or maybe they're just better at putting on a show.

"You look wonderful," Karen says.

"No, but you do!" answers Ellen.

"Nothing a month straight at the gym wouldn't fix," adds Irene.

"What a good idea," says somebody's husband.

All the babies are decked out in new clothes. They nurse. They burp and spit up. We marvel at their gorgeous fingers and toes, their smiles. We all "ooh and ah" at one another's bundles.

"Is little Jake's head always so floppy?" asks Karen.

"Not always," I say, a bit defensively. Quickly I change the subject, asking about their new home. No response.

"What does his doctor say?" asks Ellen, showing genuine concern. She and Karen gather around.

I don't answer immediately. An awkward silence follows. Ellen and Karen glance at one another uneasily. I just can't bear to enter into a discussions about Jake's deficits with this group. Fortunately, at this moment, someone passes around a tray of sweets, and the topic of conversation shifts again.

This is not easy for Jim either. We are on the verge of exhaustion. The stress of Jake's health challenges are taking their toll. We just don't know enough yet. But we're not ready to talk about it here. This is not the place to share our terror about his future. I wonder if we are so burnt out because we are older than most of these people. Even though I am feeling isolated at home and most of these women are also now around to talk to during the day, it would be an enormous stretch to connect with these joyful peekaboo players. After the pleasantries, Jim and I make our escape, eager to return to safety. In the privacy of our own home, of course, we are developing routines and take great pleasure in our little son, even though without the baby's smiles and emerging personality to respond to it is a challenge to sustain the energy that parenting requires. His repertoire is so very different. Much more limited.

One morning, one of the women in the group calls to suggest she and I get together with our babies. I make excuses. I don't give her much information about Jake —there's still not much to tell. I hedge, letting her know I appreciate the call, but that Jake's medical appointments make it hard to schedule visits. In truth, I am barely able to endure social times with friends and family I know well. Intimacy with relative strangers is beyond my reach right now. There's just too much worry storming through our lives.

Later that summer, I briefly recapture my former life as a busy union staff representative. First, I join a couple of conference calls from home dealing with the potential merging of my union of CBC radio producers with a bigger organization.

It is fascinating work, involving considerable strategic thinking. Normally, I love this kind of debate. Some days later, Jake has just fallen asleep for his afternoon nap and I am midway between stripping the bed and myself, throwing in a load of laundry and jumping into the shower. It's a mad rush to get the basics done and, maybe, read part of the newspaper before Jake awakens. When the phone rings, I dash into the living room, clad only in my tatty navy socks.

I am invited to attend a gathering of union people the following week. While we develop a game plan for the meeting, I am struck by how absurd my situation might appear. We finish off the conversation and, of course, I say nothing about being caught in my dressing gown (not even!) at four o'clock in the afternoon.

As I arrive at the meeting the next week I notice a familiar smell, that curious mélange of cigarette smoke and aftershave that means business, and Jake and I are greeted warmly by colleagues. I know that a lot is at stake for our members but at some point during the conflict-laden discussion, it strikes me that the foremost—and largely ignored—labour is the human birthing process. The impassioned debate I am part of that afternoon is quite clearly about protecting turf and territory. While I know the terrain well, today I am unable to connect with the macho strut of certain players.

I realize that being a new mother requires the precise opposite of strutting aggressively. Notwithstanding the intrusion of Jake's coterie of health professionals, he and I are meant to be suspended for a time in a very private realm, a place where nature and hormones call the shots. The contrast with the bluster before me is just too great. I am relieved to scoot home when it is over and resolve not to venture back into my old world again until I must.

4

Jakey's Hungry

AT THE SAME TIME as I have been trying to find help for our family, now and in the future, another story is unfolding in Jake's life.

Once home from the hospital, he continues to take the nipple often. Mostly I sit with him inside the house, usually perched on the living room couch. The window is just at eye level, facing south, and a fair amount of light sifts through the trees. I can see the comings and goings on our street as Jake sucks peacefully for hours at a stretch. On warmer days, we set up on the covered balcony at the front of the house. I leaf through baby care books and magazines, letting Jake feed whenever he fusses.

Our midwife, Vicky, visits every second day. Her objective is to help Jake establish nursing and also to check his weight. This aspect of postpartum care was an important reason why we decided to have a midwife as well as a doctor. But neither the midwife nor our pediatrician is pleased with Jake's progress; in these early days at home, he gains only a couple of ounces, which causes some alarm. I am puzzled, since he seems to suck, sleep, pee and poop just the way the baby books say he should.

Nursing is not easy for Jake. His suck is "lazy," Vicky says.

We want to avoid switching to bottle-feeding, if possible. Vicky shows us how to hang a bottle around my neck with a shoelace. It contains precious breast milk, expressed earlier. A clear plastic tube is laced gently from the bottle into the side of Jake's mouth so he gets a double dose when he sucks. The theory is that by adding a small amount of extra milk while he is feeding, Jake will be encouraged to suck harder and eventually latch on with gusto.

Jake is about three weeks old when we have our second appointment with the pediatrician. She is a tough-minded woman in her early sixties. "I saw babies die of starvation in Africa," she says. "That will *not* happen here." She is very stern with me and directs us to the nutrition clinic at Hospital for Sick Children. She minces no words: "This is an emergency."

Once more, Jim and I click into crisis mode. We are good at this, both of us team players from way back. Unfortunately, the physician's manner has left me feeling—not for the last time—that I have really screwed up. After all, I can't even feed my own baby. Can there be a worse sin?

The doctors at the feeding clinic are more compassionate. They insist that we use baby formula—at least temporarily—to fatten Jake up. We worry about nipple confusion, meaning that the baby learns to prefer the bottle because it takes less sucking effort, a common reason breast-feeding fails to establish. But this does not even register on the doctors' list of concerns. They're talking about our baby's survival. They do agree, however, that we may continue using the feeding tube, rather than a rubber nipple, to get as much into him as possible.

We spend a terribly intense week devoted entirely to getting Jake's weight up. It is a constant occupation, day and night. I feed him on the breast, then try to "top him up" with more milk I've already expressed. Next, I hand Jake off to his father. Jim feeds him with a wee tube dipped in a baby food jar, now filled with breast milk or formula. He places the tube, along with his meaty little finger, gently in Jake's mouth. Jake sucks, swallowing the sustenance he so desperately needs. We sleep in shifts, a few hours at a time.

After a week of this feeding marathon, we line up at the crowded clinic. Chairs are littered with tired, anxious parents, babies in tow, waiting to see their doctors. The scale shows that Jake's weight is up almost one pound. The doctors say he is now "out of the woods" and congratulate us on our hard work. One hurdle overcome. Yay Jake!

For three very full months, Jake and I continue to struggle with nursing. His difficulties are not something we anticipated. Our friends schlep their babies everywhere, the mother's breast providing sustenance, comfort and continuity. I just assumed we would do the same. I had imagined that Jake and I would have peaceful feeding interludes, mingled with occasional crying or, at worst, colic. Instead we experience intense scrutiny when he is at my breast. A lactation consultant is necessary. But it feels very intrusive.

"Is he latched on properly?"

"Can you feel his suck drawing the milk?"

"What position are you holding his head in?"

"Here, let me lift the pillow closer to your breast."

I feel like a pretzel or some oversized Gumby toy, with big boobs. Push me, twist me, I'm made of modeling clay. Eventually we'll get it right and Jake will thrive.

There's no down time; all my actions are calculated, diet and exercise, just to make this nursing thing work. I'm doing everything I can to help him feed but it isn't enough. I feel worn out. "Do I have enough milk?" I wonder. "Am I too nervous to produce what he needs?"

"No," the experts assure me. "Your milk is fine. But we have to help little Jake learn to suck properly."

Back from our trip to Ottawa and Montreal, I'm holding the fort at home while Jim is away for three weeks on a language course. We had planned for it before Jake was born, when I still thought a "wash 'n wear" baby was in the offing. Neither of us wants to stay in Toronto long-term, but Jim needs more proficiency in French for us to return to Ottawa.

Without his help in the evening, the tasks involved in keeping our little boat afloat are more daunting. I feed Jake, clean up the kitchen and living area and try to keep myself reasonably well-groomed among the poopy diapers and dishtowels. I take Jake outside in the fresh air whenever possible, once during the morning and again in the afternoon. One friend shows me how to wheel the stroller up and down sidewalk curbs gently to induce Jake peacefully into his afternoon nap.

I'm scouring baby care books to find infant stimulation ideas. I dangle a small black and white soccer ball from the top of the stroller to encourage him to reach up and bat at it with his hands. I place a mirror by his head, perching it carefully to the side of his face so he can see the "other" baby. It concerns me that my sweet, peaceful boy doesn't seem to notice any of the accoutrements I rig up for his stroller and crib.

Early in the week, I take Jake to our by now regular appointment at a breast-feeding clinic. I park several streets west of the hospital so Jake and I can enjoy the sights. It's a nice summer day in the city, not too hot. I can smell the fresh fruit and vegetables that waft from small grocery stores on our way.

The breast-feeding expert is a gentle and tenacious man with a lovely sense of humour. He knows how to motivate mothers to continue nursing, without injecting a lot of guilt into the mix. As he weighs Jake like a pound of butter in the bowl of his shiny metal scale, the physician encourages me to persist. He explains how I can supplement Jake's feeds with infant formula introduced through a tiny tube taped to my nipple. This is slightly more complex than the midwives' system, and definitely harder to set up while holding the baby.

I find that this method takes an inordinate amount of dedication—or, perhaps, sheer bull-headedness. I'm exhausted and my confidence is flagging. Not only are the women I know committed to breast-feeding, it's practically a bloody political stance. I never noticed this before. Plastered on the door of the pharmacy is a poster that says, "Breast Milk—Baby's Birthright."

"Yeah, so hang me for treason," I think, as I go in to purchase baby formula for the first time. "He's only getting it through a plastic tube, not a bottle."

Breasts and nurturing. Mothering. I wanted to be a "real" mother, whatever that was. To have patience and breast milk overflowing. I know what a mother is supposed to be—the mothers in stories are quiet spoken, all-giving and only roar to protect their children. This feeding business is supposed to be easy, the most natural thing in the entire world. Instead, I'm blubbering and, frankly, turning into a nervous wreck. At least on the inside. I pull it together for all the appointments but my internal dialogue is not pretty. Jake is already two months old and I'm not exactly glowing with the joys of motherhood.

My relationships with the health care professionals we encounter during these early weeks vary enormously. The pediatrician who worked with starving children in Africa is a no-nonsense type, very stern. We do not hit it off. I feel under attack from her because Jake is experiencing such difficulty nursing and I am reluctant to bottle-feed. But her urging that I cease to try to breast-feed and merely use any means to increase my baby's weight goes against conventional wisdom and the advice of the specialist at the breast-feeding clinic. Such powerful guilt trips are usually saved for women who have fallen prey to formula manufacturers' propaganda or those judged too selfish to give a baby its birthright, mother's milk.

My God, what if Jake and I never bond? Why the hell can't he just nurse like all the babies I see in the park with their perfectly relaxed mothers? How can I be a real mother if Jake isn't constantly attached to my breast? He needs sustenance and love. What's wrong with me? I even have a newfangled nursing bra. It's white with big black polka dots, designed to provide visual stimulation to the newborn child. If only Jake would learn to love the bra's contents!

I spend hours reading all those damned nursing books. I'd like to slug Sheila Kitzinger, that mammary maven! Not to mention the mothers at the annual picnic hosted by the midwives' collective. Wee ones are practically swinging from their mothers' tits. My tears well up just watching the proud papas and mamas strolling among the trees with their perfect children.

One evening, after a particularly discouraging day while Jim is still away, I am grateful for a dinner invitation at the home of Jake's godparents, Hinda and David. When I arrive at their door loaded down by three canvas bags and Jake bundled in his infant seat, Hinda quickly senses that something is amiss.

Soon we are all sitting together on their living room floor, tubes and bottles of various sizes strewn about us. Hinda has the Sheila Kitzinger nursing bible at her fingertips. David is helping me to position all this persnickety equipment so it works properly. Laws of gravity and volume—I knew I shouldn't have skipped grade eleven physics!

I sit on the carpet, my back supported against the couch. A small bottle of milk is set above me on the arm of the sofa. A very fine tube dangles from the bottle down to my breast, where Jake is cradled in my arms. First I must suck lightly on the tube to get the milk flowing. Then Hinda threads the tube carefully over my breast and into Jake's mouth, to encourage him to start sucking. This is meant to motivate him to work harder so he'll get additional breast milk, that maternal gold. We look like some kid's project for the grade six science fair.

Then a new point of view emerges from the sidelines. Mira, their three-year-old daughter, comes closer to inspect. She looks at me. She looks at her parents. Then she looks at baby Jake and listens to him cry. "Jakey's hungry," she tells us, with the absolute certainty that only a small child can assert.

That's it. The end justifies the means, I decide. Not only has Jake been bestowed with a wonderful new nickname, it is time for him to drink from a bottle. Three months of breast milk (not to mention a fine selection of his mother's copious tears) have passed his lips. Enough is enough.

Jakey loves his new bottles of infant formula and starts to chub up in no time. But he is still not reaching the milestones described in the baby care books I read so voraciously. Still no smiles. He's also not yet holding up his own head. I am quite anxious about my own ability to mother. Is this happening because I can't nurse him properly? The hardest part for me is not getting any response from my baby—even a little smile would go a long way.

At fourteen weeks, Jake and I are back at St. Joseph's Health Centre to see Dr. Mehta, the neurologist. He is to assess Jake's developing reflexes every couple of months. He holds up my floppy little boy and bounces his pudgy, sausage feet on the desktop. Jake is doing his best imitation of a rag doll for the good doctor; his legs dangle loosely, revealing little muscle tone. Dr. Mehta is considerate, choosing his words carefully.

"He's a lovely boy," says Dr. Mehta.

I am silent, listening intently.

He opens a manila file folder stacked neatly on his desk. He takes out a large, gray sheet that resembles a photographic negative.

"These are the results from your son's CT scan, the one taken at Hospital for Sick Children," the doctor says. "It's too soon to know exactly what the calcifications in Jake's brain will mean." This is the first explanation we've had since receiving that disconcerting telephone call about brain abnormalities when Jake was just eight days old. Dr. Mehta shows me the marks on my son's brain that may mean limits to his development.

He waits patiently as I make a few notes in the notebook I now always carry, and tries to assuage my fears. Then he schedules further tests, including an EEG, for the following week.

I pack Jake back into his Snugli and set off for home, struggling with my worry. I stop for a glass of fruit juice at a bakery with an outdoor patio. Jake is asleep, tuckered out from his afternoon performance, and seems to enjoy the shade of the restaurant's awning. But as I sip the refreshing drink, my mind continues to race. The combination of fresh air and exercise, usually so healing, is not doing the trick today. I'm tempted to ask the waitress to add a shot of vodka or rum to my drink.

Energetic people are striding along the sidewalk only a metre away, separated from us by a low, black iron fence but their footsteps and laughter may as well echo from another planet. Locked in my own private waiting game, I try to reconstruct Dr. Mehta's exact words so I can pass them on to Jim. And where is that winning smile the baby books promise at six to eight weeks? Why does Jake's head continue to bob about like a dashboard ornament?

Waiting for test results is its own special form of torture. But what choice is there?

A few days later, Jake and I are walking with my friend Ruth in a park near my parents' house in the suburbs. We have known each other for many years and somehow ended up doing similar work which has brought us closer together of late.

It is a pretty day, lots of late afternoon sun and the new sea-green stroller glides easily along the path. Suddenly Ruth notices Jake move in a strange way. His body goes tense for several seconds, then relaxes. I pick him up quickly, as if the act of pulling him in close could stop his suffering. But my touch makes no difference. Once again, Jake's entire body is frozen taut, his face caught in a frightful wincing expression.

"Why is Jake's body so rigid all of a sudden?" Ruth asks.

"I don't know," I say, terrified by how scrunched up his face has become.

"I think he might be having a seizure," says Ruth.

We fly back to the house and conscript my elderly father to drive us all down to St. Joe's. From time to time, Jake's face contorts wildly, his limbs jutting akimbo. Fortunately, Dr. Mehta is there. I fumble with my wallet at the emergency desk, trying to sort the many hospital cards I've acquired in the last three months. They admit Jake on the spot and we all settle uneasily in the waiting room.

I feel like I'm going to jump out of my skin. I realize quickly that I need the mild anti-anxiety medication my family doctor has prescribed for emergencies. Ruth drives to my house, forages through our medicine chest and returns a short time later. The medicine takes the edge off and I'm better able to focus on Jake's condition.

Jim is still away. I need him with me for this crisis. Ruth stays overnight with me; we tell the nurses she is my sister so they allow her to be in Jake's room. My parents drive back home in the early hours of the morning, only to return to Jake's bedside the next day. Mark, in whose home we were married and now Jake's honorary uncle, also joins our little vigil. Jake is very important to him, perhaps because he has no children of his own. Jim leaves his course and makes the twelve-hour drive back to Toronto. He arrives the next morning, exhausted and worried.

Jake is having more seizures which cause his face to contort and his limbs to go stiff. His bottom lip juts out each time his body jolts into freeze-frame. Doctors administer powerful medications like valproic acid and phenobarbital. Jake must stay here for a few days while hospital staff observe him. "What is his schedule? How long does he nap?" the doctors ask. They just don't get it. Jake doesn't have a set routine. We are rocking along from crisis to crisis.

I wonder if Jake can feel the seizures. They look so violent. Does it hurt? Is he suffering? The staff suggests that seizures are like an electrical storm in the brain and that he can't feel them. But how do they know, I wonder? I dash home and pull out every book in the house that might give some clues, and reread the information package the epilepsy foundation sent to us.

While Jake's hospitalization is necessary, it also carries unexpected perils. Every medical student in the joint seems compelled to examine him and identify his abnormalities for us. One found it necessary to tell me that Jake's testicles might not be formed properly. We do not enjoy watching our baby being poked and prodded in the interests of medical science. It feels like an invasion of my own body, although I'm not the one sporting the latest intravenous-wear on every limb that can provide a rich enough vein.

Once Jake stabilizes on a particular anti-seizure medication and can return home safely, Jim hopes to finish his course in Quebec. Our experience these last few days has been harrowing; I feel completely out of sync with the rhythm of the world. Although it's hard to admit, I am scared to be left alone. I would rather not be solely responsible for our son at this point. Only a few short months ago, I was criss-crossing the country by airplane, visiting CBC radio stations from coast to coast on union business. But now I'm in uncharted territory. While I understand Jim's desire to salvage what he can of his language training, I am angry at his choice of priorities. In the end, I agree to soldier on for another week, with Ruth nearby and my parents on call.

In the weeks that follow, Jake has appointments for many other things. He is almost sixteen weeks old and, in spite of all the tests at St. Joe's, scheduled for another series of invasive tests and neurological exams. We line up again with the uneasy horde at the Hospital for Sick Children downtown, waiting to see specialists in feeding and development. I now know every elevator, coffee stand and women's washroom by the main street level entrance.

One day, Jim and I meet with a new neurologist at the Hospital for Sick Children. He examines our son, who is now just past the four-month mark, and expresses concern that Jake tends to stretch himself backward, almost touching his feet with his head, his body forming the shape of the letter C. He looks like an excellent candidate for the Cirque du Soleil. This is puzzling since he is still not able to hold up his head or smile responsively.

It is obvious to Jim and me that we are dealing with a smart, highly skilled but somewhat aloof physician. He orders a magnetic resonance imaging (MRI) scan for Jake. This will take an accurate snapshot of Jake's brain and provide doctors with very detailed information about our son's developmental abnormalities. "There's normally a nine-month waiting list for this test," he says. "There are only two MRI machines in the city."

"You've got to be kidding," I say, losing patience with the whole damned exercise. Do we really have to wait nine months to hear the truth about our son? But we are having to admit to ourselves that Jake's condition must be very serious to warrant this level of urgency. We sit in shock, clutching Jake and his bulging diaper bag.

What in God's name are we meant to do?

5

Finding the Light

JAKE SOMEHOW gets his MRI soon after that but we haven't heard the results when, in spite of his medication, his seizures rocket off the meter. Again we rush with great apprehension to the emergency department at the Hospital for Sick Children. It seems filled to capacity. Much later I am holding my son in one of the stuffy examination rooms off to the side of reception. As his little body jackknifes from a seizure, I hear my name called from somewhere out in the corridor. Jim is standing at the doorway, gesturing for me to join the white-coated figures huddled to one side of the aisle. I motion back that I cannot leave Jake alone.

Moments later, a nurse slips past me into the airless institutional room. A doctor we have never seen before beckons for us to approach. He appears impatient. I settle Jake with the emergency ward nurse and make my way into the noisy hallway. I am somewhat alarmed to see that the doctor is flanked by five eager medical students. Their white coats belie the innocence of their fresh, young faces. The doctor practically rounds them up with his clipboard and prepares, it seems, to hold forth. My heart lurches into my throat.

"Your son has a rare brain condition called lissencephaly," says the doctor. He is curt. It is clear that he is addressing his entourage as much as Jim and me. We still don't even know his name.

"What does that mean?" Jim asks.

"It means your son will be severely retarded both physically and mentally and the prognosis for his life span is very guarded, " says the physician, rather mechanically.

"Excuse me?" says Jim, his disbelief apparent.

"I have the results of your son's MRI scan right here, I'm afraid," says the doctor. "Your own neurologist will discuss it with you further."

It is the Friday before the Labour Day long weekend. We are unlikely to track down "our own" neurologist for several days. This unknown physician has just delivered tragic news in the middle of the crowded public hallway of an emergency department.

The doctor and his entourage move on to their next case. The corridor feels like it's spinning. There is a clanging noise coming from an empty bed that is being wheeled past us. It is an eerie sound, naked metal touching metal. I feel utterly jangled, as if we were caught in rush hour crowds. My husband takes my hand and we go back into the room where Jakey lies. Jim holds him close to his heart, singing to him softly. We do not speak.

Lissencephaly. We have never heard this strange word before. One of the underlings who stood at attention out in the hall digs up a medical text for us to search through. There is a single line about lissencephaly, a simple definition, plus the note that typically, information about this rare brain disorder is gleaned from autopsy data. No one knows why this brain deformity occurs.

"They used to think these kids had cerebral palsy," says the intern. "It's only with the MRI that we can detect the extent of your son's abnormality."

"Uh huh," I mumble, still in shock. It doesn't seem possible that Jake won't survive. He's my baby, the one we have hoped and planned for.

I am stunned by the diagnosis but I am also quite livid. How dare they reduce my son to one bloody line in a medical text! What do they know of his perfectly-shaped head, his fine blond hair? What kind of clown tells parents that their infant will die, in a situation about as dignified as an amusement fair midway?

One more time, Jim and I go home leaving our baby in a hospital. That evening, we call in the troops. The library at Sick Kids is closed for renovations. Where can we get more information about lissencephaly? My sister-in-law, a family medicine specialist, promises to ask a researcher colleague to do a search of the literature. Computer-literate friends agree to search the internet for material.

The following afternoon, someone tracks down an article in a medical journal. It deals with the neurogenetics of lissencephaly. At least it's in English but the news is frightening. The author is conducting a study of babies born with lissencephaly. So far, he has about sixty in his sample group, mainly from the United States, a few from Canada and Mexico. Most of the children don't live past a couple of years. They aren't able to sit up. They aren't able to walk and not one has learned to speak.

The human brain is bumpy, covered with hills and valleys. This means there is an enormous surface area that allows for the storage and processing of the complex information that governs the body's higher functioning. Jake's brain is smooth. We are told that his brain stopped developing somewhere between twelve and fourteen weeks after conception. Lissencephaly shows itself in seizures and in low muscle tone. This explains his problems sucking and swallowing and inability to hold up his head, even at five months old. It also explains why he didn't tuck his head down when I tried to push him out of me.

I feel like someone just kicked me in the stomach. I can barely get a breath. My mind races, scenes of the last several months parade wildly through my mind. Jake's cries, seizures, his struggle to nurse. All in all, a pretty poor quality of life lies ahead for Jake. Jim is stoically quiet, but I can see that he too is shaken.

All the same, getting a diagnosis after months of uncertainty provides some kind of relief. It feels a bit like finally fitting all the pieces together in a complicated jigsaw puzzle. At an intellectual level, at least, some sense of order has been imposed on the chaos our little threesome has experienced during the last several months.

Still, it is hard not to feel singled out. I cannot stop thinking, "Why me? Why my son?" We must be in shock, but having to focus on Jake's day-to-day care keeps us going. One morning follows another; there's no "off" switch to this particular roller coaster. We will have to keep chugging along. My family doctor suggests I pick up a best-selling book called *When Bad Things Happen to Good People.* I can see it would be a great help to people more religious than we are.

Shortly after Labour Day, my friend Jane gives me a stress busting therapeutic massage. While she is attacking the knots that have staked a permanent claim to my neck and shoulders, I describe our last visit to the emergency ward at Sick Kids. She is appalled.

"For heavens sake, Miriam, it's a children's hospital," she says. "They can't be allowed to train future physicians like that." Jane knows that the hospital has a patient advocate, a kind of ombudsperson and encourages me to set up a meeting to investigate the way Jake's diagnosis was delivered.

I summon up my courage and make an appointment the next day. Fighting for oneself is never easy. It goes against the grain to make trouble, especially when your child still needs the best care this hospital and its staff can offer. But my sense of justice is strong, my outrage stronger still. There may not be a right way to tell a family that their child will die, but there is certainly a wrong way.

I see the patient advocate a few days later. She seems friendly enough and has an air of intelligence about her that I like immediately. She first asks how my son is doing. Then she asks me to describe in detail the incident I mentioned on the telephone.

"Well," I said, "that brute of a resident gave us Jake's diagnosis, including the probability that he will die soon, in the middle of a corridor. All in front of an impressionable herd of junior ranger med students!"

I am on the verge of losing it. No, I am losing it. She listens carefully and does not try to censor my language or anger. I am almost in tears, reliving the awful moment.

"Sounds rather cruel," she says.

"It was. Not only did he drop this bombshell in a public place, but it's one hell of a teaching example, isn't it? Why wouldn't he take us somewhere private, where we could process this news?"

"Well, that obviously wasn't uppermost in his mind. What do you think should happen now?"

"Before or after he burns in hell?" I ask. She smiles, just slightly.

I can sense from her demeanour that she is genuinely compassionate. "You have every right to tell the doctor that you found his conduct appalling," she says. "Why don't you write a letter?"

That weekend, while Jake is still on the ward, I lodge a formal written complaint with the hospital administration. I name the doctor concerned. I also ask that the hospital institute training programs to ensure that no other parent receives devastating news in such a callous fashion. Most of all, I want an apology.

I never receive a response.

After the relief of the diagnosis comes the shock. I had believed that a child born in 1990, with whatever difficulty, could be taken care of, made whole. Women of my grandmother's generation might say, "I had eight and I lost two." I certainly didn't expect that to happen to me. I ate well, exercised, and didn't smoke. We had a competent midwife as well as an experienced obstetrician. I had wonderful prenatal care and lots of birthing support. Yet my boy isn't healthy. I dredge up harrowing scenarios from the pregnancy, like needing urgent dental work when a filling came out, or slipping on the ice one evening outside my office building. I was swept off my feet by the crowd until someone stopped and helped me to my feet.

It isn't until the hospital genetics staff speaks with us that I am convinced Jake's condition wasn't caused by something I did. One of the counsellors is particularly helpful. She helps me to understand what an absolute fluke this occurrence is. She draws endless diagrams of genetic coupling, reminiscent of grade thirteen biology class. Lissencephaly occurs in one out of three hundred thousand births, most often unexplainably. I begin to let myself off the hook. What has happened is nobody's fault. Rather, it is one of those things that just happens in nature. An act of God, some would say. You can't even buy insurance to cover it.

To realize that the combining of chromosomes is nothing more than a crap shoot is rather humbling. I grew up believing that I could control a lot of things in my life but with Jake, all I can control is the kind of care that he gets and how much pain he is put through.

It also strikes me how differently Jim and I react to the scientific information. This particular chromosome lottery is our shared endeavour. But my emotional response is a strong sense of failure and self-blame. After all, it was on my side of the bed that the pregnancy and baby books were piled high for months. Jim is distressed by Jake's condition but it doesn't seem to shake his very foundation as a person, as a man. I keep functioning because I must. But inside, I am shattered.

I find a therapist, a psychiatrist, fortunately covered by the provincial health insurance plan, to help me unravel the complex layers of feeling I have about Jake—the hurt, anger, sadness, and joy. Working through it all is not an easy manoeuvre. Once a week I tromp off to her office, keenly aware of the sterility of spirit that engulfs me. It seems to breed in the hospital. I often walk long distances in the fall air just to clear my head before arriving for my appointment. In addition to the emotional work, with her medical knowledge she helps me to decipher the complex scientific articles I am reading about lissencephaly, genetics and the brain. I need to understand as much as I can about my son's situation.

Through all of this Jim still is rather quiet about his own feelings, perhaps too disappointed and concerned about Jake to open up much. This is also his natural stance. He and I recognize (and occasionally bristle at) how we process emotional material in very different ways. Still, I am worried about how little he seems to be processing the emotions that go along with this meat grinder of a situation. One morning, before he wakes, I make a couple of phone calls to his brother and to a friend. I ask them to draw Jim out, something I seem unable to do effectively just now.

Sometimes, I feel sorry for myself. It seems impossible to let go of the dream that Jake will be a normal, happy little boy. There are so many storybooks I hoped to read him. What about teaching him to ride a bicycle? Months—even years—of anticipation are hurled out the window. I feel cheated. What did we ever do to deserve this?

And what about our dreams for Jake? In the middle of one long autumn night, I remember the name I rolled over and over on my tongue before my son was born. It would have sounded simply marvelous at the end of a news broadcast: "For CBC Radio, this is Jacob Daniel Edelson in Jakarta." Or it might hang on a shingle at his labour law practice. Better yet, I mused during that long night, the Jake Edelson Trio would cut a compelling jazz CD.

Sometimes I just rage. I smash pillows with my fists, giving voice to the unspeakable sense of loss I carry. The depth of my anger rivals only the sorrow unearthed at the other end. I think about purchasing a punching bag to hang in the basement for those nights that sleep is something only other people do. I need to channel my outbursts of feeling in a way that won't hurt anyone, including me.

Some moments are more reflective—just plain sad. Grief comes in waves, often when I least expect it.

One afternoon I leave Jake's ward in search of fresh air and a cold drink. I call my friend Hinda from a nearby restaurant. As we talk, I lose it. I sob uncontrollably into the phone. Hinda, who knows me well, urges me to jump into a taxi and get out of the hospital for a while.

"Jake will survive without you for two hours," she says. "You need a break, Miriam. Now."

She's right. I hang up the drenched receiver and grab a cab outside the emergency department. Traffic is gridlocked. I sit in the taxi, which barely moves an inch, for what seems an eternity. The driver is making small talk about the humidity, a smog alert, the Blue Jays' win the night before.

This I can't stand. I have to move, walk at least. As I jump from the vehicle, leaving the surprised driver with a five-dollar bill, he calls out "Lady, come back. It's starting to move."

"I can't," I say, "My son is dying." Silence. The man just looks at me.

"I'm sorry lady. Hey, take your five bucks," he offers. But I just keep running, propelled by sheer adrenaline.

When I stop running, I have to face my fear that I am too selfish for this challenge. What if I cannot truly love my son—and what kind of mother does not feel total love for her offspring? I feel terribly exposed, as if a stranger had turned over a rock and seen my awful, mean-spirited underside. The feelings hidden there are not pretty.

Mercifully, all these different feelings quickly give way to concern for the more immediate challenges Jake faces. It's almost as if my psyche is protecting me. It won't allow my mind to focus on these thoughts for long or they will crush my soul.

By late September, Jake is still in hospital battling pneumonia and the powerful seizures that rock his brain. Watching him closely each day, waiting at his bedside for better news, I realize I need to start swimming again. Feeling all tied up in knots makes it difficult for me to perform on demand as a responsible, calm parent. I cannot have the necessary dialogue with the doctors and nurses if I'm totally overwrought. Even a short workout will help to keep the panic at bay. I can walk over to the downtown Y in just a few minutes.

I meet an acquaintance there. "How's motherhood treating you?" she asks me innocently. My carefully constructed façade suddenly crumbles. I'm babbling that Jake is in hospital with pneumonia and serious neurological problems, tubes attached to his arm and nose, and so on. I'm suddenly unable to trot out pat responses to this friend of a friend, though we don't know each other well. She insists that we sit down, gets us each a cold drink from the lounge and we talk for a while.

She puts me in touch with a family who also have a developmentally delayed son. He lives at home with his family and a younger brother. I speak on the phone with his mother a couple of times, comparing notes about feeding positions and what kinds of stimulation work. I am, unapologetically, a greedy sponge for information. We also talk about the advantages and disadvantages of keeping one's child at home and confide some of the emotional responses typical of mothers in our situation. These are not always the most generous or pretty.

Honest, heart-to-heart talk is so refreshing after months of dealing primarily with professionals. I have so many questions. I need to hear another parent who, like me, is coping but can still express fear and disappointment. I don't want the evasive answers professionals give us. I want the truth. I don't care if it's ugly, or mean.

I love Jake and will help him grow into the finest boy he can be. But to survive as a whole person and as his mother, I need truth. Frankly, I don't want to sedate or censor the outrage that swirls through my being and gives me the energy to pose tough questions. Jake is *not* the child I planned to give birth to. That child was well. That child would have come home with me after two days in hospital, and we would have built a family together.

In hospital I feel I have to show, above all, that I can cope. It is not okay to sound upset. I sometimes feel I mustn't let my guard down or they might start treating *me* with medication. From day one, neither Jim nor I found the medical staff particularly responsive to our queries and we're not exactly shrinking violets. Mothers know a lot about their children. Parents have valuable insights to contribute to their child's treatment plan. But we must have the whole truth about his condition. It is the false hope—not the reality—that debilitates us. Talking with another parent is a welcome change. We inhabit the same psychological landscape and I feel less alone. These connections are helpful beyond measure.

One morning while Jake is asleep, I walk over to a bookstore and resource centre for parents. Entering the shop I feel slightly apprehensive. I am so much less certain of my objective than when I bounded into bookstores during my pregnancy. *Then* I had simply devoured whatever information I could find about my changing body and our baby's growth.

Today I look around the shelves, taking in the huge number of titles. There sure is a lot of advice out there. Books about different age groups, ethnocultural practices, hobbies, diseases, fourteen distinct psychological approaches (and then some) to raising children—all have space in the store. But there is no section of books on babies who are dying.

Eventually, I find a small paperback called *A Special Kind of Parenting*. It speaks to me. What a relief. The introduction talks about discovering your child has a disability. The author says she realized that she and her husband had a choice. They could deal positively with their daughter's situation together or let it tear them apart.

I find some solace in these words because the author acknowledges her less than saintly reactions. This is tough emotional terrain for any mother to wander in. The author writes about the sense of loss a parent may feel and explains that with a disabled child, the feeling may resurface throughout the child's life. Typical milestones like college, marriage or grandchildren, may not be possible.

She also suggests that learning to balance conflicting feelings can be harder than losing a loved one altogether. It is not a one-shot experience; you cannot just get over it. You have to revisit the multi-layered issues over time and grapple with them again and again. Armed with this insight, I head back to Sick Kids to renew my vigil. Over time, my attitude toward Jake's condition begins to change. Gradually, I understand that I don't have to focus upon his flaws. Maybe the medical approach forces comparisons that are not helpful. The anatomically-correct child is not necessarily perfection incarnate. Besides, that's not who I've brought into the world. Whoever this tiny boy turns out to be, he is mine. My heart, like a flower opening, begins to embrace his personhood differently. Something inside me is shifting, slowly but perceptibly.

He is mine and his being amounts to more than a cold diagnosis or prognosis. I am his mother and I have a choice. I can stomp out the primal instinct I feel to protect him—which would essentially mean bowing out as his mom—or I can look high and low for ways to interact with him. I make my choice. Yes, Jake is going to die. But while he is alive, I want to keep myself tuned in and close to him physically. I want to have every possible bit of closeness with him.

What do I learn when I stop raging at his diagnosis? He doesn't know about reaching his arms out and touching things. When I put something in his hand, he doesn't grasp it. I come to see that Jake is a little boy who will not go out into the world; we have to bring the world to him.

And he does begin to respond. At first he had vision problems; his eyes didn't track properly. But after a while we notice that when he sees coloured objects or hears birds chirping, he chuckles. In fact, he loves it when light shines brightly in his eyes. One day when he was very tiny, I laid him on a towel in view of the window in the washroom while I was drawing his bath. All of a sudden he started to giggle. This was unusual, indeed! When I moved him out of the sun spot, he stopped. So I held his face up to the window and he smiled again.

Since then, the two of us have mastered many games together involving light. We play with flashlights and glittering mobiles. I tell him adventure stories by the window—"Mr. Sun" is the other main character. Jake's smiles always fill my heart with joy. They are an affirmation of life and a wonderful reminder of words from the Book of Ecclesiastes in the Bible: "The light is sweet to the eyes."

6

No Heroic Measures

WATCHING ONE'S INFANT wage a losing battle with pneumonia is alarming. Jake is four-and-one-half months old. This is a new crisis. His high fever won't break, his breathing sounds like a rattley old automobile engine that can't quite turn over and we are back in Sick Kids. Jim and I remain near, trying to comfort our son. We hold him, patting his chest and back lightly to help keep the mucus moving. An intravenous line attached to the fleshy part of his hand serves as the gateway to his complex, flawed system. I can see his red seizure medication and antibiotics travelling up the line into battle with the infection.

Such a small person alone in a big, metal hospital bed. Often, I climb in with him just to hold him close, to make him (and me) feel safe. The nurses show us how to roll up blankets to support his limp neck and to tie him into an upright position in a little sling to help him to breathe more easily. Jake's lungs, nose and throat are quite clogged with mucus. Keeping him comfortable is a challenge.

We learn to use the suctioning equipment that the nurses employ to quell the mucus flow. Wielding a very fine tube, we reach up through his nose and down into his lungs. This is very hard at first, but it gets easier (for us) as time goes by. Jake does not seem to be suffering. But to say he looks at ease would be stretching it. His little body resembles a pin cushion as IV's are moved every couple of days from heel to scalp to hand to arm and back again.

We bring children's music tapes for Jake to listen to. If nothing else, "Baby Beluga" and "Skinna-marinky-dink" cheer *us* up. He does seem to like hearing the melodies and rhythms played on the Walkman, tucked in next to his pillow. Listening to cheerful music also helps time pass for the rest of us and brightens up the hospital ward.

I do not usually stay the night. It makes more sense to snatch what little sleep is possible at home. Setting off for the hospital every morning is now my job. Occasionally, friends or family come by to see the baby and handle the devastating news about Jake's condition in their own way. The company helps combat the inevitable sense of alienation that seems to accompany a long stay in hospital. Still, I fully expect to bring Jake home soon—for good.

One day the nurses move us into a room with a four-year-old boy named Nicky. One of his eyes appears to be missing. His limbs look normal, but they are jumping at random in skittish movements and he makes odd noises. I feel frightened. Is this what's in store for Jake? My fear fades gradually as I watch Nicky and his family cuddle and play and I begin to feel a kind of acceptance. Nicky is so full of life and personality. Each day, the nurses encourage me to talk with his mother, Frances, about her family's experience as if they know that Frances and I belong to some special club, the mothers of disabled children. She tells me what it was like caring for Nicky at home, how difficult it has been to manage her marriage, her job and also care for their two other small children.

Now, after several medical procedures, Nicky is living in a small group home not far from the family's home. Safehaven, as it is called, is a wonderful parent-run cluster of group homes in Toronto. When the provincial government started pulling out of institutional care for severely disabled children in the eighties, these parents lobbied and organized, raising funds for residential and respite care for their kids. In the house, each child's room is unique, decorated with colourful posters and teddy bears. Parents are involved in their child's care along with professional staff. Families are welcome at all times in the facility. Sisters and brothers come and play and enjoy meals there; they help choose their sibling's clothes and remain intimately connected.

Back at the hospital, Nicky is never alone. Members of his extended family take shifts, keeping him comfortable and amused. One night Frances' younger sister and I order a pizza. We are playful and irreverent, letting off steam together. We can almost forget that we're whooping it up in a dingy institutional room. We learn from Nicky's high-spirited entourage to make tapes for Jakey with messages from members of our family, interspersed with cheerful kids' music.

Also inspired by the involvement of Nicky's family and friends, our friends encourage Jim and me to go away for a weekend while they watch over Jake. We eventually tear ourselves away for a day and take a drive to one of our favourite haunts, a small town where we can explore the craft shops and look at pottery. The day is clear and sunny, unusual for this time of year. I enjoy the feel of stoneware in my hands, feeling its strength. Material from the earth, hewn by loving, capable hands, seems to ground me. But we are so drained by the worry of these last several weeks that Elora offers me less comfort than usual that day.

Jim is tired and seems distant; he seems to take refuge in his thoughts. We have been so other-oriented in these months, little energy between us except to jump from crisis to crisis. Still, the beauty of the fall day is refreshing and I begin to feel hopeful in the crisp country air.

This time, Jake's hospital stay stretches to almost two months. I feel powerless, and the doctors' actions only reinforce this. Other staff make an effort, but the doctors call the shots. Their supreme authority rankles. When we are again to meet the neurologist assigned to Jake's case, it must be at a time convenient for him even though my husband is still at work. Fortunately, Hinda happens to be visiting and she comes with me.

The physician is sitting at a round table in one of the small rooms behind the nursing station. As usual, I feel trepidation as we enter the room. I introduce Hinda and we sit down uneasily. He tells us that Jake's case of lissencephaly is severe. Hinda—more in control at this point—peppers him with all kinds of questions about Jake's feeding, his muscle development and prognosis. The doctor explains that further exploration will be necessary before he can provide details with any certainty. End of meeting.

They must take lessons in being aloof, I think to myself, but at least he had the decency to sit us down away from the hustle and bustle on the ward. I take a deep breath and we return to Jake's bedside, silent and shaken. Jim arrives later in the afternoon and I tell him about the meeting.

Through all the ensuing tests and procedures, we ask that the physicians consider letting Jake die a natural death. It becomes clear that this is not a path acceptable to the medical authorities. In fact, Jake's doctors carefully avoid any discussion of this issue. Gentle dying, accepted and welcomed, is apparently not part of their mandate. Nonetheless, Jim and I persist. We feel the need to at least talk through this issue with them. In one meeting with this same neurologist, we each try to raise the possibility that Jake be allowed to die gently, without pain. Now he is clearly suffering a great deal from the pneumonia that ravages his tiny body.

"I have nothing more to say," says the doctor. "This meeting is over."

I have rarely seen my even-tempered husband so angry at another human being.

The nurses put us in touch with the palliative care team at the hospital so that we can at least talk about the possibility of letting our baby go peacefully into that good night. We learn that we can ask that only pain control medication and water be administered.

We are learning another new language, every discussion bringing the critical questions more sharply into relief. As Jake's parents, we cannot claim objectivity but Jim and I are not persons unacquainted with reason. The powers that be, however, do not acknowledge our right to engage in a full discussion about Jake's treatment, not even to sit down at a case conference with our son's entire health care team. We don't even know if there is a team that meets all together at once. Always, the doctor's word carries. End of story.

For me, the crucial point is that Jake should not be in any pain. Jake deserves parents who can face reality. We do not expect a miracle cure. The diagnosis is final and we will not put him through futile, invasive procedures.

Aspiration pneumonia is the most common cause of death for babies like Jake. Food particles and fluid get sucked into the lungs because of the child's inability to swallow and digest food efficiently. An infection develops which, in such fragile infants, is often fatal. The design flaw Jake was born with carries its natural consequence—death. Under no circumstances will we allow Nature to be plucked from the driver's seat.

We put a Do Not Resuscitate (DNR) order on Jake's chart, once we feel we know as much as possible about his condition. Jake will receive every available care to make him comfortable but if he stops breathing, we do not want him put on a resuscitator or tubes installed in his trachea. If his heart stops beating, there will be none of those heart-jumping paddles that TV emergency room doctors brandish so valiantly. As his parents, it is our ethical and legal right to make this choice. It is a heart-wrenching, sad decision but we remain convinced that this is the most humane treatment our son can receive.

For weeks, before and after our decision, Jim and I need to talk almost constantly about this. Our friends and families offer their support, making us meals and taking part in hours of tortured conversation after kids are put to bed. We look at all the angles, medical and legal, trying to ensure Jake the best possible care, with the least amount of pain. Terms like "heroic" or "extraordinary" measures begin to punctuate our ordinary conversations.

It doesn't look like our son will ever be able to eat normally. He is having difficulty breathing. Two small clear plastic tubes are stuck up his nose and down into his lungs, because of the pneumonia. His seizures are still violent and the medication has not yet wrestled them into submission.

When Jake has been in hospital for close to nine weeks, we are faced with another difficult dilemma. His doctors, representing three different specializations, decide to conduct a feeding study. They strap my six-month-old baby into a chair that is connected to a surreal-looking machine which crams his mouth with substances of various textures, one at a time. An occupational therapist watches to assess what particles Jake is able to swallow. Often, he gags. It is like watching an evil robot torture my child. I feel so helpless.

The technician insists I sit with her behind a glass partition, away from the monster machine. When I see Jake struggling to breathe, a goopy blend of pablum and tears dripping from his face, I want more than anything to burst through the glass and whisk him away from this horrible place.

Of course, I must contain myself. I am not allowed to comfort my son during the study.

It is soon obvious to the physicians that Jake will never be able to coordinate his breathing and swallowing sufficiently. As a result, they make plans to install a gastrostomy tube directly into Jake's stomach. This will allow baby formula and fruit juice—as well as his roster of medications—to be pumped straight into his tummy. Another surgical procedure called a fundal placation is also scheduled. This, we are told, will make it impossible for Jake to bring up undigested liquids from his stomach back into his lungs.

Neither Jim nor I are comfortable with the doctors' orders. We debate the appropriateness of both procedures. Our view remains that Nature should be allowed to take its course. It is disturbingly evident that Jake will succumb to his condition at a young age. Does it make sense to employ such vigorous medical intervention when he is likely to die anyway? We ask to speak with the person in charge of coordinating Jake's care, if such a person exists. It doesn't happen. Life on the ward in a teaching hospital is hectic. Various medical personnel rotate around, assigned cases for a couple of weeks at a time. After so long on the ward, we've been through several sets of bright-eyed young interns. Jim and I persist. We ask Jake's pediatrician to assist us in wresting back some control over his treatment plan. "It's strange you know," I tell a former colleague, "but this circus makes the legendary CBC bureaucracy seem highly functional."

Finally, my brother Jeff, a respirologist associated with St. Michael's Hospital in Toronto, is able to arrange an appointment for us with the staff bioethicist at Sick Kids. Just getting this meeting has involved jumping through an amazing number of hoops.

Dr. Lynch meets us in a boardroom in the hospital late one Sunday afternoon, far from the frenetic activity on Jake's ward. She offers us a glass of water and asks us about the traffic, that favourite Toronto icebreaker. I appreciate immediately the sense of decorum that she instills in our conversation. It dawns on me that we may finally have an honest exchange about Jake's life, instead of one fraught with ruffled feathers (on both sides).

"What kind of treatment guidelines are there for a child like Jake?" we ask her.

She pauses, but does not break eye contact with me. "We cannot willfully cause the death of any infant," she answers. "A child may die naturally from his or her medical condition, and parents may draw the line at certain procedures that would artificially extend their child's life."

She is knowledgeable and firm. Jim and I both appreciate her direct approach, free from the all-too-familiar snarl of power and position. Nor does she hurry the discussion. We speak about long-term care options and the way many parents become distanced from their children who are in residential care. "Often after several visits," Dr. Lynch explains, "parents will retreat gradually, usually depending upon how responsive they find their child."

We nod, trying to appreciate the dilemma. This is the first time the question of institutional care for Jake has been raised. I cannot imagine allowing my little boy to live beyond my reach.

While the discussion is very tough, meeting with this compassionate bioethicist is truly a watershed. We are forced to open our minds, to analyse our ethics as well as our emotions. Setting appropriate limits for Jake's treatment is, to say the least, a grueling process. Sometimes, there is something reminiscent of the rabbinical tradition in this exercise, as if we are debating the finer points of Talmudic interpretation. Jim and I are on the brink of exhaustion and tears punctuate almost every exchange. At other times, evaluating the practical repercussions of each proposed medical intervention is like walking through a play on the chalkboard before one's team takes the field.

Fortunately, Jim and I discover that we share a secular worldview that permits us to agree on most things as we explore the various possibilities, although this proves quite arduous. Our partnership has never before been put to such a test.

My brother is highly critical of Jake's medical team for not taking the time to involve us directly in crucial discussions about his treatment. On Jeff's advice, we ask for a meeting with the chief gastrointestinal surgeon at the hospital, before agreeing to any surgical intervention whatsoever.

This senior physician meets us in his office. He explains the two procedures scheduled for our son. We are told that Jake cannot be a candidate for a group home without a G-tube to make his care manageable. The only alternative, it seems, is to take our baby home, feed him by mouth until he either drowns in liquid he should be drinking or gets another case of (likely fatal) aspiration pneumonia. In effect, it would amount to killing our own child. We cannot fathom this. The thought of Jake gasping for breath in my arms, unable to get the nourishment he needs, is more than I can bear.

We are eventually convinced that a feeding tube cannot be avoided. But we draw the line there. There will be no fundal placation, no tinkering with his imperfect digestive mechanism. The stakes are high, because changing our minds would mean having to open Jake up a second time.

After all the soul-searching and tears, our minds are made up. There is a point in any crisis where one develops a certain clarity of mind. Jim and I are now there.

On the day of Jake's G-tube insertion surgery at the end of October, my sister-in-law Jean makes the trip by train from Brampton. We have become closer since my son's birth. She has described Jake and his challenges to her grade school students. At their church, she tells me, there is a group of close friends who frequently include Jake in their prayers. I appreciate her devotion to our child and the strong sense of family that brings her to Toronto this day. In the cafeteria, we gossip and trade stories about the family. It hits me like a ton of bricks: her children are at school in Brampton while my seven-month-old son, too, is being outfitted to leave home, to go out into the world.

"It's too soon, damn it!" I tell her. "Why couldn't he just be all right? Is that too much to ask?" Jean waits patiently until I finish raging.

"Let's go check for news up at the nurses' station," she suggests, nudging me out of my momentary despair. We finish our snack and head upstairs.

The surgery has gone without a hitch. The feeding tube is inserted, making it easier for Jake to get the sustenance and medicine he needs to survive, for a time.

"Little man," I tell him once he's back up in his own bed, "I love you."

7

Belleville or Bust

IT IS EARLY OCTOBER 1990, not long before Thanksgiving. Once again, Jim and I are waiting in the neurologist's office at the Hospital for Sick Children. Jake is still on the ward, somewhere above the room where we sit. The doctor tells us that Jake might need to live somewhere other than our home. For a brief moment, I'm afraid I might throw up right in his office. I need to run from the room.

Of course I don't. There's nowhere to hide in a hospital; even the bathroom is not a private place. I try to remain composed. It is hard enough to get information around here—especially from anyone in authority—without me showing signs of cracking when it comes. I've learned something in two months here; any attitude other than gratitude is frowned upon. A mother's emotion, particularly anger, is often dismissed as hysteria.

And no matter how shattered I am, we must continue caring for Jake, to camp out at his bedside each day, do everything possible to soothe him. I can't walk away from my baby just because he has plastic tubes stuck up his nose. We have found a way to cuddle him, even when an intravenous line is attached to a different appendage every time we turn around. Day by day, I am growing into my son's mother. To the cleaners and nurses on the ward, I am "Jake's mum." When I get up in the morning, that is what propels me to his bedside. Whether I am ready or not, a huge responsibility has been bestowed on me.

The finality of the diagnosis—and prognosis—sinks in and some of the initial shock subsides. Now we must turn our attention to seeking a placement for Jake at a public facility. Our pediatrician encourages us to think about what each of us needs; what do I need, what does Jim need, and what does our son need? It is becoming increasingly obvious that little Jake needs the kind of twenty-four-hour nursing care we can't provide him at home.

I'm a working woman and have neither the resources nor (truth be told) the temperament, to stay at home full time. Jim and I have always agreed that he would be a better primary caregiver for our children in their infancy but it makes no sense for either of us to quit work. We investigate the support available to us if we keep our son at home. None of the daycare programs I visited early in my pregnancy are able to accommodate his needs. Some of the waiting lists we're on have places for children with disabilities, but not for kids with Jake's complex nursing care requirements.

We learn that limited home nursing care is available through various agencies. The social workers at the hospital think we could cobble together between twenty and forty hours per week. Even if that could be stretched with ordinary babysitting to cover most of our time at work, nights and weekends we'd be on our own. Nor is it clear that such a schedule would be the best thing for Jake. Public home care programs, moreover, are highly vulnerable to government spending cuts and continuity in staffing is unlikely; these factors have profound implications for the quality of care Jake would receive.

One of us would have to coordinate the various therapies and medical appointments Jake requires, including neurology, respirology and care of ordinary childhood ailments. In addition Jim and I would need to procure the equipment and supplies of medication Jake needs on a day-to-day basis. This mission is daunting, certainly. More important is our concern that he receive the kind of daily stimulation he needs to develop to his full potential. That remains our primary focus.

Safehaven, the home in Toronto where another little boy on Jake's ward is living, cannot accept children who require so much nursing and medical care. The Sick Kids' placement staff steers us toward some facilities for children with complex care needs; they all seem to be located outside the city. The first one we visit leaves me cold. It is large and very institutional, with peeling green paint on the walls and the floors smell of cleaning fluid and pee. The rooms feel devoid of life. Children of various ages are either in bed or watching television from their wheelchairs, even in the middle of the day. I know within seconds of our arrival that I could never leave Jake there.

Then, one of the social workers at Sick Kids refers us to a small group home two hours east of Toronto, near Belleville, called Susie's Place. The placement staff speaks highly of Mrs. Gail Bench-Grant who runs this home for "medically fragile" children, another new term for kids like our son. The next night, I call Mrs. Bench-Grant from the pay phone on Jake's floor. I tell her a bit about my son.

Since I have been reading about palliative care and heroic measures, as well as talking to anyone who will listen, I decide to ask her right away about her views on gentle dying.

"My husband and I will not allow any heroic measures to be taken to keep Jake alive," I say. "How would you handle this?"

"Yes, I understand," she replies. "That is your decision. Other children have lived here until they died of natural causes. My staff do everything they can to keep the children comfortable until their time comes."

I like her immediately. It is obvious, even over the telephone, that this woman speaks truthfully, that her years of experience give her both a knowledge of the children's needs and a respect for their parents. We agree that Jim and I will drive out to meet her and see the facility a few days later.

The next day, Ruth, the friend who first identified Jake's seizures, swoops down to the hospital like a mother hawk fetching her young. She's come to pluck me from the jaws of despair. I am holding my son in my arms when she arrives.

"Get ready," she says. "We're going to a meeting."

"I can't," I say. "Jim is working tonight and I need to stay with Jake."

Ruth is having none of my Florence Nightingale routine. "Grab your coat, Miriam. You're getting too isolated for your own damned good," she says.

We settle Jake back into his bed. I kiss him on the forehead and tell the nurses I'll stop back later in the evening. Ruth and I set off on foot for a meeting between trade union people and community activists. We listen to the panel and ensuing discussion. Initially, my head is elsewhere, but gradually I am able to concentrate on the issues at hand. I see in the audience Leo Panitch, now a political science professor at York University. He was my thesis advisor a decade ago and we have remained friendly over the years. But I have not told him about Jake's condition. I didn't know how to broach the subject. I've been careening along the crisis track with Jake for months. Reaching out is difficult.

At the break, Leo greets me warmly and asks how I'm enjoying motherhood. He knows, from the years I was his student, that children were always on my personal agenda, no matter what else I might do in life. I tell him briefly about the events of the summer and Jake's weeks at Sick Kids. Leo puts his arm around me and we find a comfortable bench outside the lecture hall. While the meeting reconvenes, we speak together quietly.

"Why didn't you call?" he asks gently.

"I couldn't," I say. "After Jake first came home and the CT scan showed brain abnormalities, I wanted to talk to Melanie. But it was so hard to know what to say." Melanie, his spouse, knows about children with developmental disabilities from her profession as a social worker and policy analyst.

"Miriam, you know she'd love to talk with you," Leo says.

I tell him, haltingly, that Jim and I now have to decide whether Jake can live with us at home. Leo tells me about one of Melanie's colleagues whose son lives at home, but for whom residential care might be equally or more appropriate. He urges me again to call Melanie and explore the issues.

On this autumn evening, my focus is a million miles away from debates about class and capital. I am just a mother worried about losing her son. And I am grateful that the bond between Leo and myself can include concern for my son's future. Once again, I am glad that my reserve has cracked; as so many times before, I am strengthened and reassured by the response of someone I had not felt I could confide in. Choosing to place one's child in a residential facility goes against the grain, not only at an instinctual level, but also in terms of the current trend to close down institutions and move people with disabilities into care at home. The taboo I feel is enormous. In a way, Leo's response gives me permission to consider all the options, to make a decision about our son's future that is informed and responsible. I resolve to call Melanie the next day.

The political discussion in the next room is breaking up. I thank Ruth for bullying me out of my self-imposed exile and slip back to the hospital to kiss my sleeping boy goodnight.

I call Melanie from the phone in the hospital corridor the night before we go to see Susie's Place and we develop a detailed list of questions for Gail about her group home.

It is named for one of Gail's children who, like her mother, adores babies. The children live in a sprawling, one-story white brick home across a pasture from Gail's house in the country. They spend the day in a large, colourful room with lots of toys, fluffy pillows and special medical equipment. The room has windows on three sides and all the high-tech machinery cannot spoil the sunny atmosphere of the nursery. Photographs of the children hang proudly on the wall just inside the main entrance.

We learn that Gail has raised nine children, six of whom are adopted, including one profoundly disabled daughter who died several years ago. She has been in this business for over twenty-five years, initially running a group home for teens with emotional problems. She later opened Susie's Place for medically-fragile infants and children. The children are usually admitted as babies and stay for their whole lives, except for those who eventually are able to move out to live with parents or in foster and adoptive homes. We learned that each staff member is responsible for two children, meeting their basic needs and carrying out prescribed therapy routines. There is a lot of shared laughter and friendly kibitzing. Every afternoon there is a music circle, with songs and colourful rhythm toys for the children to hold and shake.

The atmosphere is joyful. A canary sings in the adjoining visiting area where families may gather among comfortable white wicker rocking chairs and tables. When the bird sings, the children perk up their ears. Even the pet is part of the kids' stimulation program. A few green plants adorn the visitors' room and there are plenty of interesting objects to occupy the attention of sisters and brothers, including an antique doll carriage and soft hand-sewn rabbits.

The staff is well-trained by Gail, women of different ages, all of whom adore children. Their maturity helps a great deal, especially when a child is very ill or dies. Health professionals are always on call and night staff are trained nurses. And because Gail has herself lost a child, her degree of empathy with parents is nothing short of exquisite. The care offered to all the children is both physically and emotionally intense, and yet a feeling of hope permeates the house.

Each child is bathed every morning and dressed in comfortable cotton jersey clothing. The same person gets the child up in the morning and tucks her in at night. This continuity is important to monitoring any changes in a child's condition; charting every cough or cold is crucial to such fragile infants and children. It also helps the caregivers and children to bond. Each child is loved for herself or himself with no reservations. A twelve-hour shift is long, but the shift schedule allows for this.

Gail's spiritual connection with these children is shared by the entire facility. This is her life's work and she knows first-hand the daily emotional struggles facing parents like us.

One child in her care, a few years older than Jake, has a milder form of lissencephaly. He is able to both hold his head and sit up and, although he doesn't speak, he is able to eat solid food. Often, he is quite responsive and smiles readily. His relatively good health offers us a measure of hope for our son. Maybe with therapy and lots of help, Jake will learn to sit up too.

With this visit, we are beginning to imagine a life where Jake would live apart from us. Through our discussions, we were able to agree upon the basic principles that would govern Jake's palliative care. Everything would be done to make his life comfortable and pain free and keep him in as good health as possible, but, should his life seem to be over, no heroic measures would be taken to keep him alive. This assurance means that Jim and I would not be constantly consumed with worry about him. Peace of mind is a cherished commodity for any parent. It looks like Susie's Place might offer us that. We come away feeling that it is a good place, a special situation. It is clear that the group home is Gail's labour of love.

I remember hearing stories as a child about a relative who needed special care. Bernard, my adult cousin, lived at home with his parents. My Uncle Charlie was a doctor, a coroner, and his medical training and income helped them to manage. But there's more to it than that. Lil and Charlie knew how their son would fare in a mental health facility in the 1940's. Medications and therapies for assisting people to live with schizophrenia were less sophisticated than today. They also loved their son, despite some of the scary episodes he and the family experienced. My aunt and uncle just felt unable to place Bernard in an institution.

Bernard lived at home with his elderly mother until she died in 1985. Only then, at the age of fifty-six, did he enter a special care facility. It was the only option. My father and my Aunt Mary navigated the complex state care system to find a place for Bernard in the same facility as an elderly uncle, someone he knew.

It was primarily the women in my family who recounted this tale of love and illness across the generations. Of course, men were involved in decisions about Bernard's circumstances and in caring for him. But the texture of the story, the details and how it felt, were shared most openly among Lil's sisters and my mother.

Although (I'm told) I blasted my own mother when she first mentioned that Jake might need special care outside our home, I now understand her gentle suggestion to have been an affirmation of life—both Jake's and my own.

Back at the hospital, I am once more fully absorbed trying not to break into little pieces. A few days later Jim and I come to a decision; we will entrust Jake's care to Gail and her staff, once he is well enough to leave hospital. But awake and asleep, I hear a violent chorus of judging voices: "How can you abandon your own flesh and blood? How dare you give him away, you irresponsible bitch." And by far, the worst, "Who did you think you were fooling? You could never be a good mother!"

I know I am doing a number on myself, but something inside me has been unleashed and it is not easy to turn off. I try to make sense of this in counselling.

Neither Jim nor I is in top form. I am expected back at work in ten days. Jake's two months in hospital have taken their toll. Exhausted by the further painful decision we have just made, we must now fight a whole new struggle with another bureaucracy. The provincial health care plan does not fund institutions like Susie's Place directly; instead, money is channeled through the Children's Aid Society. Jake is our responsibility and we will make all decisions about his care. We are horrified that the CAS must be involved, with its implication, at least to me, that we would ever abandon our son.

Like most people, I have only heard "children's services" mentioned with respect to someone who neglects or abuses their child. I had no idea that the CAS was involved in care for medically-fragile infants. Before I knew Jake, I could not have described how a medically-fragile child might look. Fortunately, others could. The legislation that governs the Ontario CAS provides for what are called Special Needs Agreements (SNAs), to support children with loving parents who are not in need of protection in the usual sense but whose care needs are greater than their parents or guardians can provide. The court-related CAS interventions we read about in the newspaper have nothing to do with Jake's situation.

This doesn't mean that the process of obtaining support is an easy one. It's a positively wretched experience. Although Jim and I have been grappling with tough questions about Jake's future for many weeks, we are forced to justify again, at every level, the decision we have made.

We run into a brick wall over the timing of Jake's placement. Although Gail is ready to receive him at the group home at the beginning of November, this does not suit the CAS. Funding is not yet approved. There is a glitch no one can quite explain. Jim and I take turns on the telephone from Jake's bedside doing battle with the various authorities as the date I'm due back at work gets nearer.

I call our pediatrician. "This runaround we're getting is ridiculous," I tell her. "I'm tempted just to pack Jakey up and take him home."

The doctor insists, politely, that I shut up and listen. She has consulted a lawyer and makes it very clear that we must not take Jake home under any circumstances. "Once you have your child at home," she says, "it is assumed that you can provide care for him."

"But we've been through that already," I say. "We can't. Why on earth do they think we're seeking a placement?"

"I know," she says, urging me to be patient. "It doesn't make any sense. But if you leave with Jake now, you run the risk of getting stuck outside the system."

So Jake stays in hospital for another few days while the kings and queens of red tape try to find a way out of this mire.

The very worst part of this, for me, is that we must take our baby from the hospital directly to a special care facility. Jake has not been home since he first started sputtering from pneumonia. I long to be with my son alone at home. I want to sit with him quietly in his room, to rock him and say goodbye gently at our own pace. Instead, we must remain at the hospital where I find it hard to feel peaceful, unselfconscious. Even after two months on the ward, I feel compelled to hide my emotions in such a public place. Snapshots of parenting in crisis, and in full view of professionals, is hardly the family album we'd hoped to create.

The night before Jake's departure is Halloween. I decide that a little levity is required—or maybe we're all just getting punchy. In any event, we make a party and invite family and friends to drop by. I am determined to give him a fitting send-off. Kids of various ages are scampering about the ordinarily subdued hospital room. This has been Jake's home for two months, nearly one-third of his life. Now, little pumpkins and witches are playing tag, hiding beneath the tall institutional beds. We put up colourful decorations and share Halloween treats with the children and staff. I spike little Jake's hair up with gel and draw him a pair of rosy clown cheeks. I write "Belleville or Bust" in flaming red lipstick on his chest. He is passed from arm to arm, like any cherished baby.

The next day is a sombre one. The Children's Aid Society has finally conferred its approval. We must take our boy straight from the hospital and drive to Susie's Place. Amen.

We receive a list of the equipment Jake will need immediately. Jim goes to the medical supply store near the hospital and picks up a feeding pump, suction machine and diapers, hardly your ordinary grocery list. Some of the cost will be covered by the provincial health plan, the rest, we hope, by Jim's supplementary insurance from work.

Jim's brother takes a few hours off work to help us pack up Jake's belongings and the new high-tech gear. I am glad he's there to wait with Jake and me in the busy main lobby while Jim fetches the car from the lot around the corner.

The November day is breezy. Not so the silent people inside the car. Neither of us finds words to relieve the sense of loss that envelops us. I am sitting in the back with Jake, who is strapped securely into his infant seat. Kleenex in hand, I make sure his breathing is unobstructed and suction his mouth and nose gently from time to time. With every passing mile, I try to memorize my boy's lovely features, his big eyes and wide mouth, the sweet smell of his perfect baby skin.

Too soon, we turn off the highway and head north past stately brick farmhouses and their land. We turn left onto the gravelly road to Susie's Place much too quickly for my liking. As we pull into the driveway, I take a deep breath. I am suspended in time, for just a moment, unable to move. I look out, noticing the simple beauty of the pasture that hugs one side of the children's house. Then Gail waves from the door, ready to greet us. I step out of the car, Jake in my arms. The air is crisp. Jake gasps in response to the cool air on his face. Jim finishes gathering up the boxes filled with equipment and clothes that our son will need in his new home.

Once inside, we don't stay long. Jim and I gather around Jake's crib, trying to settle our boy in his new surroundings. Then, it's time.

I am still holding him in my arms, rubbing his head gently.

"This is something that really soothes him. I hope you'll do it a lot," I say to Gail quietly, my voice shaking.

"That's something a mother would know," she says gently.

Her words give me some comfort as I am feeling pretty awful about leaving my son with strangers. At some level, I've not yet shaken the feeling that I am failing Jake. Gail's attitude is respectful, accepting of the predicament in which we find ourselves. She doesn't judge us for deciding that this is the best solution for our child and—likely—for ourselves.

Through my tears, I know that this is a home where Jakey will be loved. It is set up for special babies like him, infants who need constant care to survive, even while they sleep. I hope my sweet boy will sleep well tonight in his new bed.

We have taken Jake to Susie's Place in 1990 after two heart-wrenching months in hospital. First we had to decide what was the best level of care for him to receive at times of crisis; a few weeks later we had to come to terms with the necessity of his living away from us. We at least had the comfort of taking him to a home where he receives skilled and loving care. Parents today, however, have an even more difficult time finding the best possible care for their medically-fragile children.

Sadly, the plight of these babies does not receive much attention unless something goes terribly wrong. If a child dies of neglect due to substandard care in a residential facility or a parent at wits' end resorts to desperate measures, there is a flurry of concern. But when things are running as they should, these children remain virtually invisible to the public eye.

During Jake's short life, I have learned a lot about how things work in my home province; families in other parts of the country face a similar situation. When SNAs were instituted in Ontario, they were meant to ensure a broad safety net for all vulnerable children and families. The system works by funneling money from the province, and ultimately the federal government, through the CAS to the agencies or private group homes like Susie's Place which provide the direct care. The CAS assigns social work support to administer the care and pays a per diem of, in 1999, between $160 and $300 a day; hospital care is three or four times as costly.

In recent years, a widespread distrust of institutions has led to a change in the philosophy of care. This has made it easy for budget-cutting governments both to reduce funding to the caregiving agencies and cut the number of SNAs and to substitute payments to families in order to purchase the services they need from a variety of professionals and agencies, many privately owned and run for profit.

Between 1995 and 1997 in Ontario, there was an overall reduction in the number of SNAs of 7 percent; the number of SNAs for infants decreased from fifty-two to seventeen, a rate of 65 percent. Very few new applicants are receiving this support. Successive provincial governments in Ontario and elsewhere have closed down residential facilities.

This raises a serious question: where and how are these infants being cared for? There is no evidence to suggest the number of such babies has diminished. In fact, advances in medical technology would suggest that more babies are surviving into childhood. Some Children's Aid Societies no longer even keep a waiting list, reflecting regional differences in opportunities for support. Many families have no choice but to manage their child's care at home with the limited assistance available through home care. Unfortunately, adequate funding and community services are frequently not in place to replace the residential care.

Individual control over services is often equated with self-determination for people with disabilities. I believe the issue is far more complex. Individualized funding is a model that is fraught with problems.

First, the families rarely receive enough money to pay for the services they need to care for their children.

Second, it is often necessary for one parent to stay at home to co-ordinate the various therapies the child needs. This "broker" role can itself be a full-time job when coupled with the child's personal care and ongoing roster of therapeutic and medical appointments. But not every family would choose, or can afford, to give up one income.

Third, as centres of care are downsized or disappear completely, the collective expertise at our disposal as a community is also diminished. This clinical expertise does not develop overnight, nor is it readily purchased from disparate agencies.

Fourth, there are complicated labour relations issues—both for parents and caregivers. The family becomes, in fact, an employer. If one considers health and safety concerns, workers' compensation in case of accident and the provision of workers' health benefits, the status of employer can be quite onerous where individual employment contracts are concerned.

These caregivers are often highly-trained professionals, including occupational and physiotherapists, nurses and social workers. The services they provide may involve significant challenges to health and safety (e.g., heavy lifting, exposure to disease, and lack of specialized equipment common to larger settings). Who pays the cost of compensation in case of accidents? Is the disabled person's home a workplace under labour legislation or workplace safety acts? What benefit plan does the employee have access to? Who is responsible for regulating training standards and evaluating performance?

Moreover, wages for home care are typically below those in the institutional sector. Total compensation, meaning health benefits and pension protection as well as wages, is far lower. As a result, there tends to be a great deal of turnover in these jobs, similar to what I experienced with Jake's home care aides during his early days at home. Caregivers working on individual contracts can be at a disadvantage too since, like any non-union workforce, neither their wages nor benefits are negotiated collectively.

The rate of turnover also compromises the quality of care provided. If the turnstile never rests, it is much more difficult to maintain services that are high quality and coordinated to meet the family's particular needs. Parents have to entrust their fragile child to a series of strangers.

Finally, I believe that the individual funding model has a built-in class bias. It makes things particularly difficult for families who do not know the Canadian system well or whose first language is not English. To access the assistance they need, families must navigate extensive government and agency bureaucracies and cope with filling out umpteen forms for an alphabet soup of programs. This requires a fairly good educational background and a lot of chutzpah, in addition to the patience of a saint. The managing of budgets, payroll and deductions also demands mathematical and accounting literacy equivalent to that exercised in running a small business.

These are all practical concerns which affect the quality of care. Even if we do not consider here the huge ideological issues raised by the privatization of health care and social services, it is clear that the individualized funding model may not be as effective as a coordinated network of services that is universally accessible and comprehensive. There may be the appearance of independence for the disabled person. But is it genuine choice supported by a web of coordinated services that are delivered by a highly trained, stable workforce? Not likely.

Where appropriate placements and/or funding are not available, the choices for many families are these: either their children live in hospital until they die, because their parents cannot cope with their needs at home; or care at home, particularly for children with severe disabilities, places intolerable burdens on parents and siblings and often seriously isolates them from usual social interactions.

These families are not a powerful political constituency. So the rhetoric of individual choice can be used to conceal the state's attempt to wash its hands of the responsibility for funding and regulating an entire web of much needed health and social services.

I can only ask, who will be left to speak for these children?

8

Jake at One Year Old

"HERE, HE'LL LOVE THIS," says Gail, plunging Jake's right hand into the middle of the chocolate-iced layer cake.

He squeals in surprise at the unfamiliar texture and looks up quizzically at Gail. He is one year old today.

"It's *your* cake," she tells him. "Happy birthday, Jakey!"

He is sitting propped up in his blue chair near the window. We are gathered around him in the playroom. Jake's eyes are bright and his wavy hair falls away from his face. He's even a little bit pudgy in the cheeks, no mean feat for someone who lives on baby formula and juice, pumped into his stomach through a tube. When I press one of the squeaky animal toys up against his chest, he giggles repeatedly.

Jake has reached a major milestone on his journey and I have driven out to Belleville to spend the day. Gail and the women who care for Jake have decorated the room and there is a lovely birthday cake, candles, and presents for him. Gail gives him a new tape player, one of the colourful ones for toddlers. He'll be able to listen to music in his crib all the time now. And he loves the light from the flash when we take pictures.

I am pleased with our visit and thankful that so much love surrounds my son, even when I cannot be there.

Because my child is not with me all the time, it remains a struggle daily to feel that I'm a mother. I think that Jim experiences this sense of loss somewhat differently, perhaps less intensely. Perhaps it is the physical relationship between mother and child that makes the sense of separation so powerful. Jim misses his son terribly but he is able to put these feelings aside more easily. For me, there is no let up.

Jake's photos are displayed in our offices and in our home—on the mantle and in the bedroom, in the kitchen and on the piano. Sometimes, in the day-to-day rush of working and living my life, I fear that we might forget him. The occasional person has even had the gall to suggest that "moving on" or "putting this behind me" would be more healthy. I disagree. I cannot conceive of excluding Jake from our lives. In fact, I am constantly searching for ways to bring him into our circle, into the hearth of our family, such as it is.

It's tough to have a baby who doesn't live at home. There's no easy way to explain it to workmates or the man at the milk store. We have noticed that people sometimes look like they are going to crumble when we tell them about our son's condition. We don't want to upset anyone or ask for pity. But not to include Jake in our community of friends and colleagues would leave me feeling desolate. Over time, I learn to tell with whom it is safe to talk about him in detail.

We are fortunate that our families have always welcomed Jake warmly. Most significantly, our decision to have Jake live in a group home facility, rather than care for him at home, is never questioned. During the days at the hospital, my mother accepted this long before I was ready to hear it. Families need to work out their own needs and search their souls. When we realized that caring for Jake at home would not be a wise decision, we were fortunate to have a genuine choice. Many do not. Fewer staff and higher caseloads in social and health services mean there isn't always help available.

In March 1991, we visit our friends Hinda and David who, with their now five-year-old daughter Mira, are spending a weekend at a rustic cabin near a lake and a small forest of snow-frosted, green conifer trees. Jake is doing well, so it feels okay to be away for a short period. After supper, Mira and I are reading a book together. She tells me quietly, "When Jakey is older, he should come skiing with us at a cabin like this."

I pause for just a moment, trying to find the right thing to say. My heart jumps into my throat, but there's no need for my words.

"It's all right if he can't walk," she says matter-of-factly. "We can carry him."

I am awed again by her ability to take in his reality so fully.

Jim's rock solid confidence endures, a strength for me to draw upon throughout Jake's life. He is a big man, but very gentle. An ex-football lineman and serious competitive sailboat racer, he has an amazing ability to stay calm in a crisis. When Jake is home we spell each other caring for and playing with Jake and doing the chores to keep the household running smoothly. I often pretend that Jake is coming home from camp. I joke with Jim that our little fellow is just stopping in to get his laundry done. I live for these moments. I put everything else on hold when he is home. Effective compartmentalization of one's life is perhaps the only advantage such intermittent parenting allows.

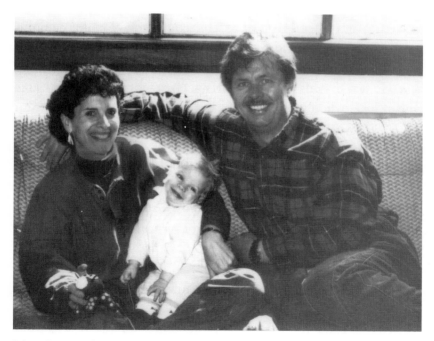

Jake at home with Miriam and Jim.

Jake arrives early one Saturday morning and will stay until Monday evening. I am taking Monday off work so we can have a longer time together. We are living in a different house now; it is on the east side of the city, not far from Lake Ontario and a shorter drive to Belleville. It feels more like home when our son is here with us.

Often when baby Jake has been at home for the weekend and I bring him back to Belleville, I stay for an extra hour and snuggle him close. He's probably ready to fall asleep the minute we get there but I need to say goodbye. And then I cry for the first half-hour of the long, lonely drive home. These are feelings of loss and sadness. Knowing that he is in the best situation possible is a relief, but it doesn't suspend the hurt that, for me, is a constant companion.

Sometimes it's hard to see other people's kids flourishing. It reminds me that my little boy isn't going to grow up. Occasionally I have acute flashes of how beautiful my son is and forget about his condition. Then I find myself imagining what he would be like if he were well, wondering whether his sweet personality would remain the same. Would a healthy child be so joyful and content? I must stay in the here and now to appreciate my son fully.

Jake's ten-year-old cousin Eric Chorostecki writes a story about him. He says that his favourite Christmas present was a visit from his cousin Jake, who has some problems and who might not live to be more than two years old. He explains that his aunt and uncle are able to feed Jake with a special machine and that he smiles at him. Eric says he can tell that Jake knows he is loved. A poem Eric wrote about Jake was later published in a children's poetry journal. Other children have since sewn special soft pillows for him, written touching poems and delivered heartfelt speeches to their classmates about Jake and his special challenges.

When we bundle Jake up for walks along the boardwalk by the lake, Jim attaches the portable suction machine to the bottom of our big jogging stroller, so we can grab the vacuum-like hose quickly when it is needed. Kids in the park sometimes stop to check him out and ask questions about his machinery. I am always careful to protect Jake's face from the wind, the way Gail has shown me. Learning these caregiving skills is important to us.

Some of the necessary nursing techniques are complicated. We give several different medications, at varied schedules through the day and night, administered through the gastric tube. We flush it through with an extra syringe of water. (His chaser I call it.) His feeding pump is on a pole like an intravenous drip. He is attached to this at least twelve hours a day and we can take it off when we go for walks or on a short visit. I also give him chest therapy two or three times a day, gently patting his chest and upper back over his lungs, to loosen the mucus and ease his breathing. We are increasingly adept at putting on the Ventolin masks that help to dilate his bronchial tubes. And at suctioning his nose and throat when he can't move the mucus on his own. If I can't mother him well by nursing him and taking him to swing in the park, I'm damned well going to do it with chest therapy!

We are now relatively proficient caregivers. For sure, there is a learning curve and the staff at the group home guides us with warmth and humour. On one visit home, Jake's gastrostomy tube falls out while I am changing him. I call out to Jim in an utter flap, "Jakey's tube fell out and there's liquid seeping out all over the change table." He races upstairs.

"Should we rush him down to Sick Kids?" Jim asks.

"No way," I say.

I do not want to spend hours in the emergency department, especially knowing how much unwelcome interest Jake's condition tends to stir among medical students. We are perplexed for a few moments, knowing that he cannot be left safely with a gaping hole in his belly much longer. In the end, we find the spare tube Gail always packs in Jake's suitcase for such emergencies and she "walks" Jim through the procedure over the telephone.

The partnership we are developing with Gail and her staff means we can "apprentice" in this special kind of parenting, without bearing the full responsibility for Jake's care. This includes emergencies from time to time, where the nursing knowledge required goes above and beyond our ability. Since even the basic activities such as feeding and breathing are so terribly complex, it is wonderful to develop patterns of caring for our son that also feel safe. I pray that further spending cutbacks won't threaten this precarious balance we've managed to achieve with Gail. My love for Jake is solid as a rock.

Every little thing he can learn to do is a gift. A few months after his first birthday, Jake begins to take tiny amounts of solid food, in addition to his formula through the tube. It's such a treat to feed him tart peach purée and watch him enjoy the pleasure of taste. His mouth puckers up and he smacks his lips from the unfamiliar sensation, as if we'd given him a lemon wedge instead of baby food. These are cherished moments.

I would still like to have a baby who can learn to say "Mommy," a baby who can wrap his arms around my neck. Jake can't do that but seems to recognize my voice when I sing to him. He knows that he is loved when he's in his Dad's arms. For any child to feel loved and comforted—and above all, to be safe—is the bottom line. I have stopped wishing he were somebody else. I am finally being able to say, "This is just who Jake is. He gives us back what he can and our job as parents is to give him as much as we can."

Sometimes, I am aware that I inhabit a kind of parallel universe. When colleagues chat about evenings spent out at parties or in restaurants with friends, the gap I feel between their experience and my own is not simply the Great Divide between those of us with children and those without. Death is always present in the universe I navigate. It sometimes dangles very close, only to be put temporarily on hold. I feel suspended, at times, in a bubble that transports me between my work life and my hours with Jake. Perhaps that is why our story is so much like one of a relationship between new lovers: all senses are heightened and one cherishes every single breath together. We are in a place apart from the bustle and ordinary cruelty of the world; a place that is inhabited by few, and truly understood only by them.

At the beginning of Jake's time in Belleville, Jim and I would take turns doing the driving when we brought him home about twice a month. One of us would pick him up and the other would deliver him safely back. We did this willingly because we wanted to spend time with our son. Then we learn that the CAS has a program for families like ours. They organize volunteers to drive children with disabilities to health appointments and other activities in the community. Some drivers ferry children from group homes outside Toronto into the city for family visits. Volunteers' basic expenses are covered and the CAS coordinates client requests with the available drivers. The first time a long-haired, single man arrives at Susie's Place to pick Jake up, the caregivers grill him mercilessly. "Do you know the address in Toronto?" "Do you know how to operate the suction machine properly?" "What would you do in case of an emergency?" Their anxiety, and absolute need to pepper him with relevant questions, is recounted to me on the telephone barely minutes later, so that I, too, can "check him out" upon their arrival.

One set of volunteer drivers nearly becomes part of the family during the many months that they transport Jakey back and forth. They arrive at the front door and call out, "We have a little package for you from Belleville." These are wonderful moments. One's sense of community broadens even further as different people share responsibility in keeping the family strong.

But now, in the early nineties, the program is moving uneasily through a restructuring meant to streamline services. Cuts are definitely on the horizon. This causes me several sleepless nights. The drivers have helped us beyond words. I am coming to realize that it is the cumulative effect of fatigue in our situation that is dangerous. Losing these drivers will leave an enormous gap, not one we can fill easily.

I try to figure out how we might mount a protest. I get names of people in the Ministry of Community and Social Services and write a couple of letters. But the line item for volunteer drivers would certainly appear innocuous at an agency budget meeting. Provincial (and federal) spending cuts have given birth to a bevy of bureaucrats wielding sharp knives.

I also approach one journalist in Toronto who writes on social issues. But this volunteer drivers issue is not really "sexy" enough to get much media play. The cuts haven't yet happened and the media are most interested in reporting tragedies that have already occurred.

And since spin doctoring is what I do for a living, I can easily see journalists retort, "What's the big deal, you're already getting practically full funding for his care?"

I wonder what happens to families who do not own cars, or don't drive at all. Or who have other children to raise and might need to stop overnight at a motel during a long drive, especially in winter weather. Most of all, I am angry that the very people—the Children's Aid and all the officials who espouse so-called family values—don't get it. This public service, the volunteer driver program, is the glue that helps keep my family—and many others—together. We did not choose these circumstances. Jake's condition just happened. We're doing our best to make it work in a way that is humane and respectful of his needs as well as our own. I would appreciate at least that much regard back from the people who create provincial ministry and CAS priorities.

On a particular weekend in June of 1991, I've planned a get-together with friends for Saturday night. When I telephone to confirm Jake's drive schedule, the CAS person coordinating the rides tells me she cannot get anyone to drive him back and forth.

I am devastated. It is so difficult for me to create family time that includes Jake. "But I've made plans. I need him to come home!" I sob.

Now I can hear the woman on the other end of the phone crying too. What a pair we are. I suppose I was just charged up with anticipation. And I know the woman feels that she's failing me. She calls back later in the evening to say they found someone to do the drive. I am reminded how much many of these workers feel for the families they serve. I feel fortunate to live in a country where such services are—at least for the time being—available.

At the end of my maternity leave, I start a new and demanding job as communications director for Bob White, the president of the Canadian Auto Workers' Union (CAW). As during my leave when I took up the reins at union meetings, I experience a tremendous disparity between my two worlds and the kinds of energy required. Union work is hustle-bustle, with a measure of bullshit and blarney thrown in. Mothering requires just as much organization and endurance, but also sensitivity and melding of self with another; hard-edge versus soft, aggression versus receptivity.

The job means a lot of travel, writing, media relations and running the powerful auto union's communications department. I also teach courses in media skills to union members. It's a tremendous challenge and very rewarding.

Nonetheless, I am having a hard time. It may be that my emotions are just catching up with the reality of Jake living so far away. Work is a terrific diversion but I miss my son constantly. Inside, I feel hollow.

When things go awry for me emotionally, there is (by now) a familiar pattern. I have trouble sleeping. Weight starts to fall off my frame. I feel extremely anxious and even vigorous exercise doesn't quite quell my worry brigade. At thirty-four, I don't yet have an adequate arsenal to battle these symptoms. Massage, exercise, talk therapy and time seem to be the most effective.

During this somewhat turbulent period, I still talk to Jennifer, the genetic counsellor from Sick Kids. She is generous with her time and keeps me up-to-date on research that helps us learn more about Jake's condition and that might assist us, should we wish to have another child.

Later that autumn, I am in St. John's, Newfoundland, gathering material for an article on fish plant workers I plan to write for the union's magazine. As I ride in a taxi to the airport, my cellular phone rings. It's Jennifer. She has located a doctor in the United States who is carrying out groundbreaking research on children with lissencephaly. She is hoping we will participate in his study. We need to send off various bits of information, as well as photographs of Jake, as soon as possible.

I know this is important work—and it is hopeful, in contrast to so much of the information we have received. More will eventually be known about this rare brain disorder. Jim and I have already agreed that we want to help researchers as long as Jake is not put through any more pain or procedures.

But at this precise moment, the call just reminds me how little power I possess. I can't change Jake's future. The finality of his diagnosis—and short expected life span—is one bitch of a brick wall. At some point in the conversation I break down, my face pressed up against the back window on the sidewalk side of the cab. It's raining outside too and I'm trying not to draw too much attention to myself.

Jennifer gently takes the time long-distance to talk me through it and I am touched by her concern for families like ours. She has posted Jake's picture on the bulletin board in the genetics unit at the hospital. He's grinning, looking almost mischievous posed in his blue chair. I thank her for the call and am certainly more composed by the time we reach the airport. The cabby, who had discretely handed me back a wad of tissues, wishes me a good flight.

This is not the only time I am overcome with unbearable sadness and anxiety. Once home in Toronto, I take steps to do some more internal work. Will it never end?

Once again, the mothering network, through my friends Hinda and Jane, leads me to just the right psychologist. I felt an affinity to her when, a year ago during Jake's long stay at Sick Kids, she came to see us as she was interested in helping us with his care.

And so begins a relationship that will last several years. Jinks (a nickname) is very helpful. She creates a safe place for me to experience the bumps in my journey with Jake. Frequently I walk in a nearby park after our sessions, trying to make sense of the tears and process of grieving I am travelling through. The journey weighs heavily upon me. Jinks helps me learn to express the fears, joys and, occasionally, the anger I feel. I learn that the whole spectrum of feelings is permitted; one needs simply to experience them, not run away. The sadness won't kill me. In fact, I shake less from the awful anxiety when I can cry or yell it out.

Not having to walk this dark road alone is an enormous relief. I learn to hold contradictory feelings in my heart simultaneously— love for Jakey and my profound disappointment over the loss of our life together. Over time, I am able to avoid succumbing to the sad-

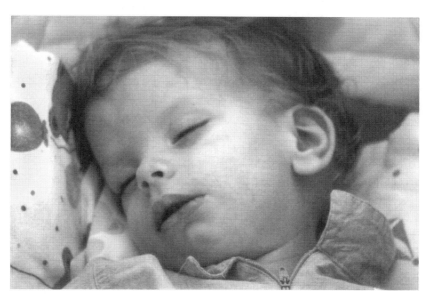

Jake naps in his crib at home.

ness. Jinks helps me to stay the course, both as Jake's mum and in my professional life.

The disparity between the two sets of demands made on me is among the issues I confront in counselling with Jinks. She helps me to devise practical solutions to the pulls in opposite directions I am experiencing—my desire for home and hearth, while also travelling the country learning an exciting and very challenging job. Like many people, I have always found it difficult to preserve my sense of being grounded, or centred, while living out of a suitcase. And yet, at least some of the time, I feel I am achieving an acceptable balance.

The CAW has an education centre for families at Port Elgin on Lake Huron, west of Toronto. The union runs a unique summer program for members, their spouses and children. Sometimes Jake can join me there. During the day while I am working, he is cared for by one of the childcare workers who has experience with special needs kids. She learns to operate his equipment and walks him in the stroller during the afternoons.

It is 1991 and in mid-August, I have *my* big day. I am completing my first triathlon in a park near Guelph. Jim ferries Jake from Port

Elgin to cheer me on. This summer, I have spent hours training, riding my bike and jogging on the tree-lined country roads whenever I am at Port Elgin. This afternoon Jake sits propped up in his stroller amid all the commotion and keeps an eye on the proceedings. First, a small, cool lake for the swim, then into bicycle gear for a twenty-kilometre ride, all capped by a ten-kilometre run. (In my case, definitely a jog.) It is thirty-seven degrees Celsius, humid as hell, and a ridiculous day for exercise of any kind. But I make it and Jake survives too. And we have the photos to prove it.

When I first took the job, I was completely frank about my son's condition and my need to remain involved in his life. Bob White was quite understanding. His view was that so long as he could reach me by cellular phone, I could work from the car on the drive to and from Belleville. Since most union conferences are scheduled for weekends, this allows me to spend a day during the week with Jake, when necessary.

Soon after the triathlon, I am in Port Elgin for meetings when I receive an urgent phone call. Jake is extremely ill. Gail says he might not last more than a couple of hours and I am terrified that he will die before I can get there. That has always been my worst fear. I am a six-hour drive away from Belleville but I need to hold Jakey in my arms right away.

Driving so far alone is dangerous under the circumstances. Jim is on a baseball vacation in the U.S. with friends, traipsing from city to city, seeing major and minor league games along the way. I call Ruth to see if she can meet me in Toronto in four hours and make the remainder of the trip with me. There's no answer at her house.

As I'm casting about for a solution, my boss calls over to tell me that he has chartered a small plane for me; a union brother will drive me to the tiny airport at Wiarton. I will fly across the province to Kingston where the spouse of another staff rep is waiting to pick me up and take me to Jake in Belleville, almost an hour away. Bob's wife will haul my other belongings, including my bike, back to Toronto. Bob takes down the names of Jim's buddies and promises to contact their spouses. We must find him and get the news to him quickly.

I am totally blown away by this kindness. The entire trip should take only two and one-half hours. I call Gail and ask her to tell Jake to hang on. Mommy's coming.

Under other circumstances, the airplane ride would have been a blast. We fly east, over fields and forests, until I see Lake Ontario in the distance. A friendly woman greets me at the airport and shuttles me right to her car. She hands me her cell phone so I can call Gail, before she reports back to Bob in Port Elgin that we're now racing west, back toward Belleville.

Jake is soon in my arms and then, very gradually, he begins to improve. Maybe he won't die, yet. He remains very pale, a slight blue tinge to his fingernails. His breathing is very shallow, his airways blocked by mucus. His eyes stay closed for long periods of time throughout the day. How can this be the perky little fellow I saw only ten days ago?

My parents are there when I arrive. They were the only ones to answer their home telephone when Gail called and, fortunately, were able to drop everything and make the two-hour trek. Later the first night my parents must return to Toronto, but their presence even for a few hours is comforting. I do not want Jake to die in someone else's arms. If at all possible, a family member should be holding him when his time comes.

For two nights and two days, and then some, I stay with my boy. I hold him in my arms and try to breathe for him. Gail shows me how to pat his body gently with a soft white cloth and liquid soap. We don't give him as much chest therapy as usual for fear that it will tire him out too much.

Jim is tracked down in a small town in the American Midwest. He calls me the first night. By then, Jake is beginning to rally. Since there isn't really anything Jim can do, we agree it isn't necessary for him to rush home. While I miss his presence, I feel very secure with Gail and the other women at the group home.

I get away for short periods of time, usually at Gail's suggestion, so I don't get too overwrought and burn out. Like anything else, there seems to be an optimal pace to caregiving. A breath of fresh air and a sandwich help to sustain my energy. I stay close to Jake for long periods of time but Gail sees it as part of her responsibility to also watch over *my* health.

By the third day, after much hands-on care, Jake is breathing more easily. He is still very weak from the virus that vanquished his system. Any infection is a danger for children like him; their immune systems are weak, and a bug that might knock another child out for a couple of days can kill them. Fortunately, Jake pulls through.

In the middle of this crisis, Gail and I become a touch punchy. Neither of us is sleeping much. We are giving Jake chest therapy, gently tapping his chest and back over the lungs. Then we check the quantity, colour and texture of his mucus. In the wee hours one morning Gail turns to me and says, "I'm a connoisseur of mucus you know." In no time, I'm on the floor laughing hysterically.

A colleague arrives on the third day to give me a ride home. His son is in the final stages of a poignant battle with cystic fibrosis. I have visited with their family in Port Elgin and we have pledged to help each other through critical circumstances. My union brother's constancy in this emergency sheds new meaning on the term solidarity.

Bob encourages me to take it easy for a while before getting back to warp speed. I need the distraction of work, but without the usual degree of pressure. Later, I see that I was naïve to think I could just jump back into work without taking time to recover from coming so close to losing Jake. Nor did I have any idea that my son's bumpy ride would become so draining for me in the longer term, diminishing my own resilience.

This, the first of many such crises in Jake's years at Susie's Place, has fueled my passion to defend his right to live in a humane setting. I am also increasingly aware of the support *I* receive; being able to count on Gail's devotion to Jake proves an enormous source of strength. Knowing that Jim and I are not alone is a huge relief indeed.

About this time, I also begin to make links with activists in the disability rights movement. I learn that one in ten of us can expect to be disabled at some time in our lives. This makes me realise that my long battle on behalf of working women with family responsibilities is linked fundamentally to issues of employment for people with disabilities. Both deal with altering the structure of work and the workplace to allow people to contribute to society on their own terms. At the end of 1992, I urge the CAW leadership to participate in a program to sensitize members and staff on disability issues.

The young man who joins our staff for a while as a result uses a wheelchair; his mother was prescribed the drug thalidomide during her pregnancy. All the same, he has been able to pursue his studies and work in a variety of settings. With the assistance of a personal attendant who travels everywhere with him, he speaks to many union gatherings.

He is able to encourage our members to see beyond the labels: a wheelchair, for example, does not have to be a barrier to an individual's work or activism. During these months, he contributes to discussions about bargaining, the economy, seniority and social programs.

The kindness I am shown by my colleagues and the progressive work I am able to do sometimes seem at odds with the burly male culture of my workplace. I write and publish an article I call "Toxic Testosterone: A Feminist Dilemma" in an attempt to make sense of my experience. In it, I admit that I was learning a lot from the self-confidence and thick skins of my colleagues but point out that they might learn from the women's movement how to move their egos over now and again, to allow other voices to be heard.

The new focus to my activism on disability issues, including finding a voice for public interventions on the radio and in print, makes me optimistic that Jake's life has meaning and that, together, we are making our mark.

One night in April 1991, Jim comes to my office to listen to the CBC Radio documentary "Mother and Son: The Story of Miriam And Jake." I had suggested to my friend Karen Levine, an executive producer with CBC radio, that we create a radio piece to publicize the sort of care Jake is receiving at Susie's Place and to recognise the work of Gail Bench-Grant. A three-part radio documentary, run over consecutive evenings on *As It Happens*, is the outcome of that collaboration. The comfort I feel speaking to a person I trust in a studio makes radio a perfect medium; my voice delivers an intimate account to an audience I don't have to look at.

I've done a lot of public speaking but never on such a personal subject. I want it to come off well—to be neither melodramatic nor maudlin. The morning of the first broadcast, I tell my new boss that the documentary is airing and that I hope the message is not too raw for public consumption. He has encouraged me to do the interview, to speak out in defense of services that children like Jake need. But I don't know how people in the union will react. Will speaking out as a mother affect my credentials? Bob's support has made it easier for me to take a risk and allow my innermost feelings about Jake and our dilemma to be broadcast across the country.

I assume the building is empty, but when the first segment ends a few of my colleagues troop in, some with tears in their eyes, to congratulate us. Speaking out bravely, forcefully, is a part of the oral

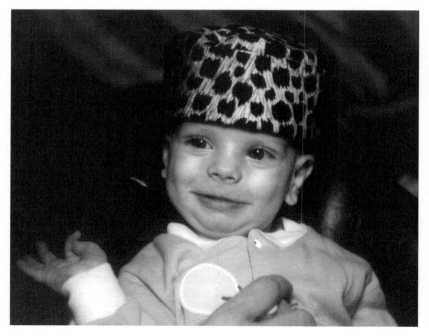

Jake plays dress-up.

tradition that marks our union's gatherings. Stripes are earned in various ways, but showing personal strength through adversity is approved. I feel good about the issues raised in the documentary and don't lose points for disclosing my feelings, after all.

Jake gives me reason to find my voice, to speak publicly about difficult issues. I cannot do this honestly without showing my vulnerability. The impetus to speak is related somehow to making my son's precarious life mean something. After all, he won't grow up to make a contribution in his chosen field of endeavour. He just is who he is. But perhaps the rest of us can learn something from his experience of the world.

A great honour is bestowed upon us a few months later when our documentary receives a media award from the Canadian Association for Community Living (CACL). All three of us travel to Ottawa to attend the banquet and receive the award, presented by Peter Gzowski, one of the judges.

Coincidentally, the keynote speaker at the CACL conference is Bob White. He and I have carefully prepared his speech and he delivers it the morning of the banquet. Unions have historically presented some difficult issues for people living in institutions. A staff member at a facility who behaves inappropriately, for example, still has the right to representation by his/her union if any disciplinary action is taken. On some occasions, the values of our legal system (innocent until proven guilty) come into conflict with the lived experience of people without power (e.g., residents of institutions). The speech offers support for people who are battling for self-determination and respectful treatment—from society and from the people who deliver the services they require.

Bob's speech also argues for appropriate and meaningful employment for people with developmental disabilities, for decent pay and benefits, but also for a new definition of what "doing your best" means. For a labour leader, so steeped in the hierarchical and competitive milieu of the shop floor, this is a huge leap.

Jim takes Jake to the dinner banquet to receive the award while I am stuck in bed with flu at the hotel. Jim speaks eloquently and is also taped for *As It Happens*. He talks about the scary prospect of diminishing resources for health care in this country. "There is no question that if we lived in the United States, Jake's enormous need for special care would have bankrupted us," he says. He holds our child proudly in his arms as he speaks and, on the radio broadcast, I hear Jake cooing into the microphone. He too must have his say.

9

Trying Again

JAKE'S NEAR BRUSH with death in August 1991 has a profound effect upon me. One thing is immediately clear. I want to try to have another child, a healthy baby. I cannot bear to lose my son without another child in the picture. Of course, Jake's condition means we harbour some fairly major fears, but loving my son for who he is means embracing the attendant hurt and disappointment, without losing hope for the future.

We know that the type of lissence-phaly Jake has is not passed on from generation to generation. His condition is in the Act of God category, a fluke which occurs in one in three hundred thousand births; there's no scientific explanation of the cause so far. The research that includes Jake's profile in its study confirms what we read in articles when he was six months old. All the same, lingering doubts persist.

When we moved from the west to the east side of Toronto, we looked for

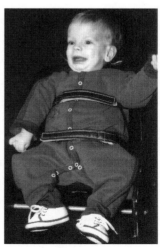

Jake in his chair, one year old.

a house where wheelchair access would be possible, with enough room for both an active child and one who will always be cared for like a baby. Jake will be longer and heavier, if he continues to survive. He will always need his specially formed plastic chairs and high-tech equipment. He is growing but will never be able to eat in the usual way.

In the end, however, practical issues are only part of the equation. We want to have a child and so we take the plunge shortly after Jake's first harrowing chute to the netherworld.

Soon after I know I'm pregnant, we learn that genetic researchers at the Hospital for Sick Children and in the United States have discovered the microscopic piece—the short arm of the seventeenth chromosome—that is missing in Jake. This means that now they can test my amniotic fluid to see whether the new baby is afflicted with lissencephaly. My workmates are forgiving of my occasionally ragged nerves, once they know the score. I travel the country with a packet of soda crackers and can of ginger ale at the ready. I am five months pregnant when we receive confirmation that the baby growing inside me is healthy, a girl, and we know already that we will call her Emma-Maryse. Emma means "one who heals" and is, in addition, a reference to Emma Goldman, the great Russian-American anarchist-feminist. Maryse is a popular Québécois name and happens to be the name of two of the fourteen young women killed by Marc Lepine in the 1989 Montreal Massacre.

I search the literature written for families with disabled children. Siblings of kids like Jake often feel they must compensate for their disabled sister's or brother's weaknesses—that they must somehow make up for their sibling's inadequacies. Also, the child may feel disappointed at not having a regular playmate. Jim and I see a family counsellor, referred by our doctor. We talk through our hopes for Emma and discuss ways to avoid the worst difficulties. We hope awareness of the pitfalls will prove an ounce of prevention.

Through our concern, it is important for us to remember that our experience as parents is not, by any means, an entirely horrible story. I have learned a lot about accepting a child who lives with a

severe disability; it also means accepting a part of myself. Tolerance
for difference is a principle that now informs every aspect of my life,
including my experience as a social activist. It fuels my desire to see
those differences embraced and celebrated in society and accommo-
dated by employers.

We all have sources of pleasure and consolation that give meaning to our lives, that we turn to in times of stress—everything from
baseball to playing the flute. I have often found solace in the beauty
of the arts. As well, I join a group of Jewish women who meet monthly
to learn about the traditions of our people. We are a diverse group,
interested in studying Judaism from a feminist, non-heterosexist
and critical sociological perspective. None of us feels particularly
comfortable in traditional congregations, but together we are exploring which parts of Jewish practice we wish to integrate into our
lives. I find a great deal of understanding and support in the group;
these women help me feel less marginal because I am an intense and
emotional person or because I tend to think too much.

While I am learning that to strive for perfection in every situation
isn't appropriate I also come to accept that nature still calls the
shots, even where medical knowledge is advanced. This also raises
the issue of our responsibility as a society. Everyone who raises a
special needs child is a pioneer. There is no map. We need to be
treated respectfully and not expected to cope alone. We are not su-
perhuman and we need help. Families touched by disability need
comprehensive and accurate information as well as social and practical supports.

During my pregnancy, we have an opportunity to consider bringing Jake back to Toronto. There is an opening at Safehaven where
Jake's former hospital roommate Nicky lives, but our son's complex
care needs are too great for them to manage. I was excited by the possibility of having him closer; it would be much easier than trekking
to Belleville all the time, especially once our daughter bounces on
the scene. The Safehaven house is only ten minutes from my office
and I can imagine taking my lunch there a couple of times of week.
What a treat it would be to visit with Jake so frequently. Because his

care at Susie's Place is above average, we can deal with the disappointment. We'll have to find another way to juggle spending time with Jake with the needs of our new baby.

Jim and I are a great team when faced with practical adversity. Our strengths are complementary. I can be quite driven—very useful in casting about to find a network of resources, for example, or generating creative solutions to problems. Jim is more placid, always maintaining a certain detachment from difficult situations. This allows him to feel in control and use what he considers to be good judgment. Jim's detachment, however, is irksome for me, just as my desire for greater emotional engagement is difficult for him. The beginning of our relationship was very different. Then, we bubbled with conversation, feelings to share and stories to tell. Perhaps we've just weathered so many crises together that we're stuck, our wheels spinning in a rut. We continue to offer one another a great deal of support, but the difference between our temperaments irritates both of us.

I hate it that this situation is so bloody stereotypical: emotional woman, logical man. Jim and I are still very affectionate, but something is missing. Time will tell but the gulf I feel is disconcerting. We plan for a birth in hospital. Our friend Jane will attend, as at Jake's birth, along with our doctor and midwife. When Jake was snatched from my body, I felt a profound sense of loss. The possibility of a normal birth is exciting and I anticipate experiencing the sense of closure that eluded me first time around.

Often I speak with our midwives of my fears for Jake once the new baby comes. It concerns me that I won't have the time or energy to remain as fully involved in his life. They have some practical ideas, like getting a babysitter for Emma when Jake is at home so I'll still have some undivided time with him.

It is important to have Jake close by during the pregnancy, and he spends many weekends and holidays at home with us. I fear that I will miss him and give him less attention once his sister is born. He's home right up until the last minute when my labour begins. We awaken one of his uncles in the middle of the night to stay with Jake while we rush off to the hospital. Later, our friend (Uncle) Mark delivers Jake safely back to Susie's Place while Emma is pushing her way into the world.

Emma is born at ten-thirty in the morning on May 31, 1992. I finally get to push out a healthy baby. Once at home, Emma's dark hair falls out, replaced by fine blond locks like her brother's. She is bright and cheerful, equipped with a powerful set of lungs. In a couple of days, the Canadian Labour Congress convention begins in Vancouver. I had hoped to take my new little bundle out west with me, but she is too young and I am still too weary to manage it. A wise colleague reminds me there will be other opportunities when my daughter is older.

I love having both children with me on these early summer days. The season is in full bloom and we walk by Lake Ontario every day. Emma falls asleep easily in her sling, enjoying the rocking motion as we walk. Jake is seated comfortably in the baby jogger, the ever-present suction machine attached at his feet. When I feel too warm, we rest in the shade on a park bench.

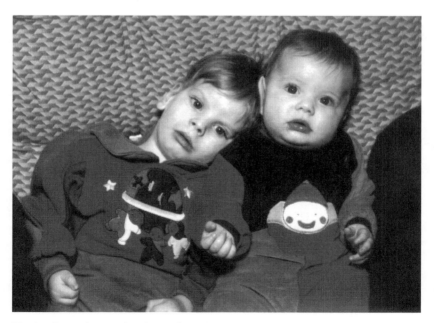

He ain't heavy, he's my brother. Jake with Emma.

Emma nurses for two months, not without difficulty. Once again, I am meeting regularly with breast-feeding experts. (I swear if we ever get a Ministry of Children's Services, this doctor should be the deputy minister responsible for breast-feeding.) Like her brother, Emma appears to have a lazy suck. This scary news evokes in me many of the feelings I experienced two years earlier while nursing Jakey. Jim and I decide to supplement Emma's feeds with baby formula. This is disappointing but I know she will not grow up to be an axe murderer because I gave her a bottle. In fact, she thrives.

Jake has a beautiful, healthy younger sister. She looks just like her brother when she wears his baby clothes but it is a different experience to care for a healthy baby. I realize that not dressing her in Jake's baby outfits is better than saving a few dollars. Like all new mothers, I am always tired and I struggle to keep my mind clear. Emma is a new baby with huge needs of her own for nurturing and mother love. I erect a dam to hold back the dark thought that any day, the other shoe will drop.

During Emma's early days, it is fairly easy to care for the two of them but when she becomes mobile it is more of a challenge—her curious little fingers find Jake's plastic tubes very interesting. Sleep deprivation accumulates for Jim and me as they awaken each other during the night. Like many families, we finally figure out that putting children in separate rooms makes good sense.

Ruth, a constant source of support during Jake's early travails, reminds me that I may need some help with Emma when she is three to four months old. At first, I resist this counsel. It is not always easy to have perspective on one's behaviour, especially when things are on the verge of getting out of hand. But she is right. Three months or so into Jake's life, exhaustion made me feel like I might come unhinged. So three months into Emma's, Jim books some vacation time. They hang out together, allowing me to escape for a swim or jog. This helps my body recuperate from the sleep deprivation of the early months. We spend part of this time at the CAW Family Education Centre in Port Elgin. I sit inside at meetings, Jim walks our daughter around. Many of the men come from fairly traditional backgrounds and, to a certain extent, the union remains a haven for burly guys fighting tough battles. One of my few female colleagues thinks it is great for the guys to see a father playing such an active nurturing role with a tiny infant.

In September, Emma and I go off to Play and Learn, an integrated nursery program for infants, the one Jake would have gone to if he had stayed at home. It is enormously stimulating for the little ones and I also hope we will meet families like ours. It would be good for Emma to know other children who have sisters or brothers with special needs. I wonder how she will react to her brother as she gets older.

Emma and I also go to Lullabies and Lap Rhymes, run by a folk singer and poet who adores children. She teaches us songs and rhymes to enjoy with our babies. Like Jake, Emma is very sensitive to sound and delights in music. This is my favourite activity with her so far. She smiles and giggles, takes pleasure in hearing my voice and tries to respond in kind. I am grateful for the chance to experience the blessings of a healthy child.

When I return to work at the Auto Workers union in February 1993, Emma is a delightful nine-month old. The usual kinds of pleasures and frustrations accompany this small, noisy package; her playful, determined personality shines through. I feel wretched leaving for work the first mornings, although my daughter seems quite content at home with her father who is now taking three months paternity leave to be Emma's prime caregiver until we locate an appropriate child care situation. I signed Emma up for various daycare programs in the neighbourhood when she was conceived but most only accept infants from eighteen months of age. The daycare centre at the school where we hope she will attend junior kindergarten doesn't begin until age two and a half. I also visit a few home daycares in the neighbourhood, but am not comfortable with them.

In a way, this search is not unlike finding a care situation for Jake. Emma's needs are quite different, but the bottom line is the same. We need a safe placement with someone who will love and respect our child, while providing quality nurturing each day. After several weeks without uncovering a single prospect, I am feeling nervous. Quitting work is not an option financially and, while I can work from home some days, I don't have a predictable schedule. Communications work deadlines are short and, when urgent issues arise, reporters can't wait for baby's naptime to a snare comment from the union.

Just as I'm starting to fret, a woman who babysits for Emma from time to time decides she would like the job. Emma knows and likes this caregiver who has also babysat for Jake on occasion. This means Jake can be dropped off on Thursday nights now and again so we can all be together for a long weekend. It's amazing how things work out sometimes, just when they seem to be heading straight into the ditch.

Jim is happy to stay home with his daughter but I know I will have to change my rather manic morning routine to accommodate a baby's needs. Reading two or three morning papers and timing my shower to catch the radio newscast isn't possible any more. What I have underestimated, however, is the way my job definition has changed, making the workplace culture even more hostile to the claims of family life. While accolades are heaped on someone available to the cause day and night, there are no points for rushing home at six o'clock to hold the baby before she falls asleep. But I still hope to juggle my way through Emma's first few labour-intensive years.

Not long before I return to work, I am asked to sit on the Ontario Federation of Labour (OFL) executive; each of the large unions has a designated seat representing women. I accept after discussion with Jim and a trusted colleague, knowing my OFL affirmative action work will be added to my regular workload. It is an honour to be asked, however, and I don't want to let down my new boss.

The first OFL executive meeting I attend, in March 1993, is out of town. It feels good to be back in the saddle in my professional life. I have something to add to the debates, including a push for affirmative action vice-presidents to be established for other equity groups, such as Aboriginal workers, people of colour and workers with disabilities. At the National Day of Protest in Ottawa that May, Jim and I carry Emma in her backpack. Free trade, plant closures, layoffs, and huge cuts in health and social services mean working people are suffering. I am proud to walk behind the colourful CAW banner. It is time to take a stand.

In the summer of 1993, the union is gearing up for negotiations with the three big auto manufacturers. Oddly enough, I had planned for my second child to arrive in the spring of 1992 so that six months before the 1993 Big Three negotiations, I would be back at work, ready to boogie. Every three years, autumn brings a ritual of intrigue and suspense. Which company will be the target? Can the plant leadership contain members' militancy as bargaining rolls out? The president is at the negotiating table and dealing not only with powerful auto giants, but with the unpredictable dynamics of member-driven bargaining teams who are connected to thousands of members in plants and offices.

None of these challenges seems to faze my boss or his lieutenants: they live for this. The Big Three negotiations are *their* triathlon.

Union staff people join reps from each workplace in downtown Toronto hotels for weeks at a time. Long hours, day and night, are spent holed up in smoky meeting rooms. Coffee and more coffee helps to fuel the lively internal debate that accompanies all major transactions at the master bargaining table. A pack of reporters camps out with us and my role is to handle media relations and organize press conferences.

At times, the dynamic between the union's chief negotiator and the companies—or the CAW teams—is akin to a ritualized dance, a highly charged tango in a smoky bar; every move is choreographed. The careers of plant and office leadership are equally at stake. As in the dance, Big Three bargaining is designed to display a powerful male strut of determination and endurance.

My daughter takes her very first steps the day we open talks with Ford in mid-July 1993. Fortunately, I am home with her that very moment, grabbing a change of clothes and giving her supper before heading out to another meeting.

As we complete bargaining with the industry target and move operations to the next hotel, I begin to question my wisdom in taking this on. The work is intense, challenging and passionate but

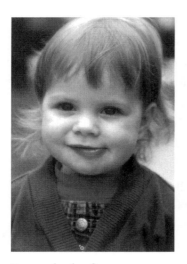

Emma takes her first steps.

juggling my duties is a challenge. Jim brings Emma to the hotel after he finishes work so I can feed and bathe her while he goes to the gym. I read her a bedtime story then he takes her home for the night. I stay in the hotel, needing to be up early for media work and meetings with the bargaining team. My stamina flags as I try to keep all the balls in the air. Gains achieved in auto bargaining, including pensions, paid education leave, and reduced work hours, have improved the lives of countless working families. But through the hard debate and protracted hours—punctuated by social relations best characterized as "Hail fellow, well met"—I miss my tiny daughter. The allure of the power breakfast is gone. My lap is too empty without the presence of Emma's warm little body at the break of day. I begin to see that it was naïve of me to try and mother her in the midst of this demanding work pace, at least, not without the support of a devoted wife.

Despite all this, most of the time I am still enthusiastic about the work. I travel a lot and, as often as I can, I take Emma with me. Later that fall, we go to a conference east of Montreal. Emma does well in unfamiliar surroundings; the union provides daycare in a hotel room outfitted with toys and trained child-care workers. I keep her fed, changed and contented at other times. But managing that, while also trying to contribute effectively to the meeting, is a challenge. There's no such thing as an on/off-duty switch in the CAW. It is a vocation, a twenty-four-hour commitment. Back at the Toronto airport late Sunday night, a small but scary thing happens; should I take it as a warning?

I have to lug our suitcase and push Emma across the roadway between Terminal 2 and the parking garage. As I lean over to put her in her stroller, I lose balance and fall on the curb. My nose begins to bleed and, looking down, I see blood dripping onto Emma's cheek and my sweater. Fortunately neither of us is really hurt. We are not far from the escalators and I finally get us to the car. Setting off to drive home, it suddenly strikes me that I will have to start the whole enterprise again the next day.

Business travel is frequently difficult for new mothers but I suspect there is added stress for me because Jake doesn't live at home. I feel strongly that I must "do it right" with Emma. On long flights, however, it just isn't practical to take her along. While at home, I am also still intent on making my weekly trips to Susie's Place. Managing the scheduling and logistics in my life has become far too onerous.

Jim tries to help out, make compromises. He works mostly in Toronto and is senior enough to have control over his schedule. Sometimes, when I am in Port Elgin for a few days, he meets me halfway to Toronto so we can perform an Emma "handover." We don't have much time for each other. We are both very involved with our daughter but I think we have forgotten how to nurture one another.

Clearly, I am reaching my emotional limit, separation anxiety overload with respect to my children. I am not completely aware of this, nor do I realize that my half-acknowledged rebellion is a healthy response to an impossible situation. One day Gail tells me that she believes my emotional energy is "spoken for" dealing with Jake's illness and caring for an energetic toddler; she thinks I need less demanding paid work. This is not an easy message for me to take in. Stubborn by nature (I'm told), it will take me a while longer to reach a similar conclusion.

The shit hits the proverbial fan one December day in 1993 during a meeting at the union's Toronto office. I am suddenly unable to formulate coherent ideas. The words in my brain run all over each other. Back in my office, I feel as if in a stupor. A colleague comes to check what kind of shape I am in. I tell him I feel dizzy and not fit to drive. Jim leaves his office to come and pick me up and we see our family doctor that afternoon. Diagnosis: a panic attack; burnout, severe anxiety and depression all go together. Treatment: time out to heal.

I apply for, and get, medical leave. Unfortunately, things get worse before they get better. Even with a potent sleeping medication, I get no sleep for four days. Getting dressed in jeans and a T-shirt takes every bit of concentration I have; leaving the house is out of the question. I finally get some sleep but my feeling that I have totally failed both at my career and as a mother are hard to shake.

It's no picnic for Jim either; I'm not exactly a joy to live with. He cares for Emma in the evenings. He's a wonderful, loving father and she doesn't suffer unduly. Soon she starts daycare and enjoys playing with the other children, climbing on the playground equipment in the large schoolyard.

I can care for Emma at home but am anxious in noisy or unpredictable situations. Life with a toddler is anything but predictable and I do not always know how much activity I can handle. Taking her for a short walk in the snow only becomes possible after I have been off work a couple of months. I feel safe reading stories and playing with her at home for measured intervals. Jim sometimes finds this scene a bit tiring. On occasion he is irritated to miss his workouts because I need him nearby.

Mostly, though, he supports me through this dark period. He encourages me to do some of the ordinary tasks that now seem risky, like making a grocery list and going to the supermarket. I force myself into a non-threatening situation by visiting the library where I can thumb through magazines and maybe even dare speak with people. Taking in a movie is out of the question for several months—the stimulation is too great. Since Jim and I have always lived very independent lives, my illness throws a wrench into our routines.

Reading and writing are the most difficult activities. My mind won't focus attention, as if my brain houses a series of post-it notes that keep flipping by. I can't stop them for long enough to read the print; it feels like too many files in my head are open at once. I learn to appreciate less challenging activities—tasks with a beginning, middle and end, like baking cookies and folding laundry. Eventually, especially if I get a lot of fresh air when out walking, I can read and absorb one newspaper column at a sitting.

In my worst moments, I feel like the character played by Meryl Streep in the movie *Sophie's Choice*, a mother forced to choose between her children. My little daughter needs her mom and knowing this has added to my already stressful situation. In addition, I have another baby (because even at four, Jake is still a baby) who can survive without me in his good care—but *I* need to be with him. In those darkest moments I have to tell myself, "My little girl is healthy and going to live. I must concentrate on making sure she gets what she needs from me." Because both my children are beloved, I feel utterly bereft.

No one should ever have to make such a horrible choice. If an appropriate facility for Jake existed near our home, both my kids would get what they need. Living with the constant anguish spawned by separation from one's child is something no parent should have to accept when it could so easily be prevented. It takes a few months before doctors identify the antidepressant medication my body can tolerate. Even with the Prozac generation of drugs, I have to deal with a variety of side-effects, which range from the sublime to the ridiculous.

Nevertheless, with all my experience of navigating the healthcare system, my foray into the labyrinth of psychiatric services is both perplexing and frightening. One dark day, a young psychiatric resident meets me for about half an hour. His response to my tale of woe is to prescribe one of the older antidepressants that I know produce significant side effects. I express my reservations and the meeting is brought to a quick halt—end of discussion. My return to the sidewalk that afternoon feels especially cold.

Our family doctor offers to see me once each week for counselling until I can be set up with another medical professional. (Jinks is away at this time, which I later call my winter vacation at Club Dread.) I eventually learn that on top of all the other issues that lead to my breakdown, I suffer from a cyclical form of depression that is worst in winter, exacerbated by lack of sunlight. I will have to take precautions in future, such as therapy with a full-spectrum light, to avoid the abyss—my own private hell.

I make progress over time. Once she returns, Jinks again helps me to understand the duality of my emotions and, moreover, to accept them. There is room, she says, to be madly in love with Jake and also to feel angry that he will never, for example, enter grade one at the public school around the corner. Over the months, feelings of anger and sadness spill out—Jake's birth, my work, missing Emma, our troubled marriage—my body and soul are reeling. I plan to start making changes in my life, to be content to be a "good enough" mother, to feel less driven and inadequate. And I want to continue to make a worthwhile contribution to society, in the labour and social movements.

In late February, 1994, I visit my parents in Florida. Before Jim and Emma join me for surf and sun, my parents and I can talk without reserve for the first time in years. They are aware that my life is in utter turmoil at work and at home. Even so, I am surprised by my father's take on my job, the job I had dreamed of throughout my career. At the ripe age of eighty, he has developed a more mellow way to measure life's achievements.

"If working for the Auto Workers is making you unhappy, maybe it's not right anymore," he says one night over supper. "You don't have to do it, you know."

I almost fall off my chair. My Marxist father, the man from whom I learned passionate ideals and my driven demeanour, sympathizes with my internal struggle. I simply have too much on my plate. Dad's recognition that I must make a significant change in my life has powerful meaning. Not that I need his permission but his acceptance that, for whatever reason, I cannot resolve my dilemma makes me feel more confident in finding ways out of it. I want to be more available to my kids and to keep myself healthy. I already exercise, but I need to live a calmer life with fewer time zone changes. Meantime, better nutrition, therapeutic massage, and chiropractic care will also help.

A month after I joined the CAW, an acquaintance quipped, "Oh yeah, and how are *you* going to handle the workaholic culture, guys one-upping each other about their heart conditions?"

"Excuse me?" I said.

"You know, Miriam, 'I had a double bypass and was back at the bargaining table in a week', one guy will say. 'Yeah, so I had a triple bypass and still walked the picket line that weekend,' his buddy says."

At the time, I could only shrug my shoulders. It's true that endurance, the sheer ability to keep going in the face of tremendous stress, is highly regarded in the union movement. The same may be true in corporate culture. That certainly doesn't mean it's good for anyone.

I return to work on a temporary reduced workweek ordered by my doctor but when it isn't possible to negotiate a more manageable schedule for the medium term, I have to move on to another job. I write an article called "The Boys Just Don't Get It" and it is published later in the year after I sign a contract with another union.

In my article I challenge the demands unions make on their employees and wonder if this culture of dedication and commitment may not sometimes be a screen for those who simply wish to escape other responsibilities. I describe my own experience:

> When I was leaving my union recently, I was challenged as to how I would act "if something were really happening," (e.g. major political upheaval). I could only answer this guilt-laden question by saying, "Someone would still have to change the damned poopy diapers!" And they would. Political struggle as an escape from the more mundane aspects of family life just doesn't cut it in my books. And I believe this narrow view of struggle has an impact on more than simply individuals. It is hardly clear that the workaholic model makes for healthy union leadership or policies.

The issues I raise will later be incorporated into some labour education programs and academic courses, beyond the CAW. Health and safety activists and women in the movement, particularly, tell me they make use of my article.

During my sick leave, my boss asks me to lunch to discuss my return to work. I don't understand. He is a tough negotiator but I have also seen him show a lot of empathy and caring during the time we worked together. I ask to put our meeting off for a few weeks. I am still under treatment and awaiting results, still too vulnerable to carry on a proper conversation with anyone, let alone my boss.

My family doctor comments, "Well, if you had a broken leg, your boss wouldn't invite you to go for a walk, would he?" I try to explain that this was no ordinary boss, no ordinary job. But she has a different and wiser perspective; mental illness carries no stigma for her. My reluctance to have a meeting reflects symptoms common in depressed individuals.

Five years later, I can see that perhaps I should have more fully disclosed the nature of the illness that overtook my life for a brief time. But back then, I was not ready to accept the diagnosis myself or to "come out" as a person who lives with depression, a condition that is intermittently disabling. I recognize now that it's a lifelong illness awakened, in part, as a response to extraordinary stresses. While it's no picnic, I now also know that I can manage it successfully. To be vulnerable to serious clinical depression is not to be incompetent or dangerous. There is little that distinguishes me from someone who, for example, learns to live well with diabetes—or any other chronic illness; we should all expect employers to accommodate us in a fair, respectful and flexible manner. If an employer decides that a worker should not remain in a particularly sensitive job, this should be dealt with by negotiation, case by case, to find an outcome that makes the most of what the worker can contribute. This was not my experience in 1994.

Perhaps, too, we ought to recognize that people who burn out are, in fact, the modern-day canaries in the mines. Workplace stress causes heart attacks, substance abuse, marriage breakdown, suicide and other health problems in all kinds of settings. If workers don't fit the mould, maybe it's the mould that should be reshaped.

10

Sister and Brother

TOMORROW, May 31, 1994, is Emma's second birthday. She is sleeping now, worn out from a day of walking by the water and listening to her Barney tape. It is the only music she wants played in the house. One night last week when she was up way past her bedtime (for a change) I reached my Barney limit. I convinced her that Eric Clapton's acoustic *Unplugged* tape is really Barney playing the guitar. She nestled in next to me and promptly fell asleep. Now two albums top the charts at our house.

We will celebrate Emma's birthday on Sunday in our backyard with friends and family. I've arranged a ride in for Jake, now four, to join the party. He needs more frequent suctioning now, so two people are required in the car. Fortunately, an elderly couple that adores him volunteers to make the trip.

At half past two in the morning, we are startled by the telephone. It is Gail. She says that Jake appears close to death. Again a virus has caused his health to deteriorate rapidly. Even with chest therapy and frequent deep suctioning, he is short of breath and litres of mucus are lodged in his chest. At this moment, he cannot muster the strength to move it. His seizures are also getting worse. The anticonvulsant medications are no longer as effective and a scan indicates constant seizure activity flashing through his brain.

I jump into the car and drive through the dark. The winds off the lake intensify my feeling of loneliness. Jim stays with Emma until she can get off to daycare in the morning. I hope like crazy that Jake won't die on her birthday.

I have never made it to Belleville as fast. It is quarter to five when I arrive at the door. Jake is lying over a wedge of foam on the low-slung bed just outside the kitchen, the spot designated for the child most in need of quick attention. He is very quiet and has hovered in and out of consciousness through the night. My beautiful son is very still. Gail says, "He is still alive, but I have not been holding him. I've just been stroking him, because I wanted to save his energy for you to comfort him." I rock Jake and suction him when he needs it.

As I am holding him, I recall that we noticed a change a month ago. For the first time, Jake was unable to sit propped up in his little chair but lay over a wedge with his head down on a pillow. He was having chest therapy, skilled hands patting his back and suctioning mucus. Piped in oxygen delivered him more comfortable breath.

That day, he needed to lie still and let the mucus flow from his body. His caregivers and I altered his position frequently, keeping his head low and elevating his torso slightly with pillows. Gravity rules. Jake was very tired and even our old standby the light game elicited no smiles. When I saw him like that, it began to dawn on me that we might be moving into Jake's home stretch.

Yet now I push aside the idea. I am so focussed on Jake's breath that the realization he might be dying lies beyond my grasp.

A large brown oxygen machine hums like the bass tone of our techno-kid's orchestra. A clear, slim tube attaches to the pint-size oxygen mask that covers Jake's face.

I hold him in my arms this early morning. A long time passes, maybe several hours. Nothing dramatic happens. The house is silent, the other children blessed with sleep. Jake remains very still. I speak to him softly, sometimes singing our songs. My mood swings from resistance to acceptance of the idea that he might be dying. "Jakey, if this is your time, just relax, honey. Just relax and let yourself go," I tell him. "You know that Mommy and Daddy and Emma love you. You are the best boy Mommy could have and I will always hold you in my arms."

Jake does not die. He holds on, a fighter with more stamina than we know. I stay with him a few days and then return to the city, drained and also moved by his caregivers' absolute constancy and regard for him.

A few days later, I again call Karen Levine at CBC Radio's *As It Happens*. I describe Jake's crisis and say, "I am a bit raw now, but it may be a good time to tell another chapter of Jake's story." She asks me to come come downtown to tape it.

I arrive the next day with a packet of photographs to show her, all taken in the last couple of years. We set up in the studio and Karen guides the interview gently. The result is another thirty-minute documentary, *Miriam and Jake: the Story of Mother and Son, Part Two*. Once again the audience response is enormous. Our program is aired again during the Christmas week "Best Of" programming. It is also one of a handful of programs to be nominated by the CBC for a prestigious Peabody Award, in the public service category.

This honour is testimony to the vital role public broadcasting plays in this country. In this intensely personal story, with the expertise of a producer and technician, the bare voice of a mother describes almost losing her son. It is a universal drama. Perhaps this public expression of my private grief can make a difference in the lives of other children and families.

It's an early fall day in 1994 and Jake is well enough to come home. Emma likes to push her brother in the large, purple jogging stroller we call the Jakemobile. Occasionally, she insists it is her turn to ride and tries to climb in too. Jake is bigger than she is now. We must be quite a sight for onlookers, with kids and a suction machine hanging off this baby jogger, a kind of all-terrain vehicle. These are the best moments—I have both my children together in the circle of my arms.

Later that year, we are getting ready for the winter holidays, the first Christmas two-and-a-half-year-old Emma will remember. Jim's family celebrates Christmas together in Sarnia, four sons and their

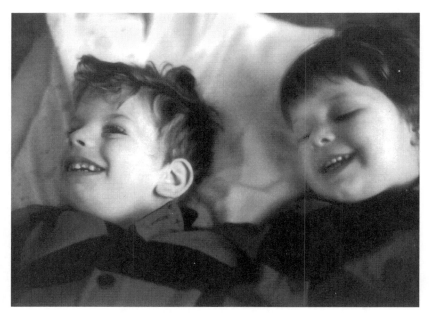

Matching P. J.'s! Jake and Emma at home.

families gathering with Grandpa John for joyful days and presents galore. But Jake has again caught a virus of some kind and is not in any shape to travel. I can't bear to be more than a couple of hours away from him when he's not well, so I elect to stay behind in Toronto and spend Christmas Day in Belleville cradling my boy. At least *I* feel safer when he is in my lap. I know that he is getting excellent care but after four-and-a-half years walking a tightrope with him, I can only feel at peace when he is nearby. Somehow I must balance my need to feel intimately connected to my son while also getting on with the rest of my life.

I have to admit that this division of responsibility also reflects troubled waters in our marriage. Family holidays are marvellous but it is no secret they can also be demanding in extraordinary ways.

From the beginning of our relationship, Jim and I have shared secular beliefs. We agreed that our children would be raised with knowledge of Christian traditions but that we would take concrete steps to impart a Jewish cultural identity. While the difference in religion is not a great chasm for us, however, the holidays tend to

trigger other tensions. As well, the dearth of natural light, the short-
ness of the days at this time of year, do not help my frame of mind.

The Saturday before Christmas, our whole family is in Belleville.
Jake's cough is quite sobering. He is again lying over his white wedge
pillow with his head down.

Gail and the staff bring Emma books and toys. After she has
cased the joint, moved all the dolls' furniture, pushed the antique
wicker buggy up and down and checked out every teddy bear in the
visiting room, she too cuddles her brother.

We usually stretch out on the carpet with Jake, although Gail has
comfortable rocking chairs for visitors. For about an hour, I lie on the
floor with Jakey face down on top of me. He is very peaceful. I love to
feel his heart beat on mine through his light fleece clothing. Jim and
I wipe his nose and deal with his endless mucus flow while Emma
looks at her books. Sometimes she plays with her father, occasionally showing Jake pictures in her books or burrowing in my lap.

Later, at home, Emma stays close to both of us. She asks me to
sing her the Jakey song, which is actually a song I adapted from Barney (ugh). Jake (that is, Mummy) sings to her, "And you know I'll
always care, even though I can't be there, I love my sister, Emma's
my sister." And she sings it back to him too, except she uses the word
"brother." It's as if she knows what the future holds, wise beyond
her years. Sometimes she comes for a cuddle, as if she's trying to
comfort us. It's a lot for a little girl to carry but, so far, she is thriving.
More and more, she speaks her worry, but never loses interest
in seeing her brother. I am grateful for this time together as a family
before we set off in opposite directions for Christmas day.

I am glad that Emma knows her brother and hope that after his
death, she will feel his presence as a positive part of her life, remem-
bering him as someone she loved, but to whom she had to say goodbye. I hope this intimate knowledge of disability and death may
enrich her emotional life as she grows, adding a special layer of empathy and forgiveness. I try to let her be comfortable with him without forcing expectations on her, making every effort to respect her
rhythm. When we visit, if she needs time to just toddle around and

play with the toys, that's fine. When she is ready to be close and give her brother a hug, that's great. When I am holding Jake and she wants to be on my lap too, we figure out a way to do it.

Often when we visit, Emma plays with Stephen, a bright and responsive little boy of about her age who lives at Susie's Place. He sits on a small cart with big black wheels and Emma pushes him around. Sometimes they have a snack together. I think for her, at ages two and three, visiting Jake means going to a special children's house filled with great toys and friendly motherly figures. What could be more fun?

From our home we say, "Hello Jake across the lake" as we look east to Belleville. At Chanukah, we light candles and call out holiday wishes to him. Sometimes when I am driving her to daycare and reach the top of the hill where she can see Lake Ontario, she will shout, "Have a good day Jake, I love you!" So far, she loves and accepts him for who he is.

I've thought up little tricks to help her feel connected to him. She helps me pick out a small toy or T-shirt to take to her brother when we visit and I always sneak in first and hide a treat or game for her in his bedclothes. She takes great delight in discovering these. How does Jake know she loves *The Little Mermaid*?

At three years old, she is beginning to grasp that Jake is different, like the character in a storybook we have read about a girl who is mentally challenged and her brother. A few months ago, after her brother had been very sick, I told Emma that Jake was feeling better. "Will he come out of his chair now, Mom?" she said. Another day she told me that he doesn't know how to talk, even though he's older than she is. One day, she asked me why her brother can't walk. Understanding comes slowly. We won't rush anything. There will be time for explanations when she is older.

The summer Emma is four, I choose a spot where she plays in the park to plant a tree for Jakey. I want to feel his presence near our home. There I'll have my two kids together, one playing, the other at rest. The park is dappled with playing children and I imagine that Jake is one of them—although *he*, of course, would listen to his mother. As the other kids retreat to their homes, I picture Jake swinging gleefully in the park, lulled by the water lapping on the beach below. At first, Emma says okay to the tree. But the next week she explodes at me during a walk to the corner store. "No, I don't want a tree," she says. "I don't want my brother to die."

In some way she recognizes a connection between the tree and Jake's eventual death, although I have never framed it this way, and refuses to accept it. I do not speak of it again. It is too powerful a symbol of Jake's mortality for her to bear at this point.

She is becoming a sensitive, articulate young person. She objects when I laugh at the things that pop out of her mouth; she is proud and sure of herself. Yesterday, after we visited Jake, she turned to me in the car and said, "Tell me how he is going to die. Is it going to hurt?" At the moment, while he is doing well, I try to reassure her as I listen to her concerns.

Sometimes we drop in on Jake at night, on our way to the cottage we have recently built on the land in the Gatineau Hills near Ottawa. The other children are already tucked in when we wake him for a

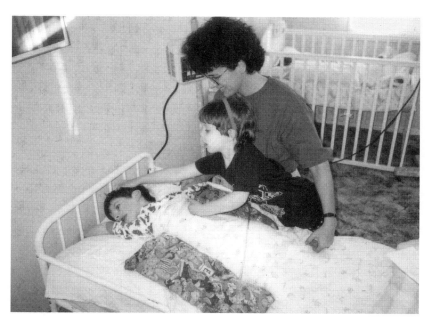

Emma helps tuck Jake in at his group home.

cuddle. If Emma hears other children crying, she goes to check on them and tells the night nurse what's going on. These little children are part of her world and she seems to understand their vulnerability without making a big deal of it. Sometimes she brings her flashlight so we can play the light game. She shines it in Jake's eyes and he smiles sweetly back at her. We sing songs and tickle him. She loves it when I sing him songs she remembers as the ones I sang to her. When it's time to go, she helps me move him back to his bed. She holds his head and gives him a little kiss before we go. Always the interaction is on her terms; this is important. She must not feel compelled to care for her brother. It has to come from her.

I follow my instinct mostly and occasionally search out professional advice to help my little girl weather the turbulence of this journey we are on together.

One of the less obvious benefits of Jake's care is that Emma does not feel jealous of the attention he receives. Certainly she misses her brother and at times this is difficult. But her parents are not totally occupied in caring for him day and night so she gets lots of one-on-one attention from us. When we visit Jake, she finds her own rhythm and keeps busy playing or colouring. She rarely gives any indication of feeling ignored. She knows the staff by name. They always offer her apple juice or some new toy to try out. I think she understands that her mom needs some concentrated quiet time with her brother and she gives me that space quite naturally, especially if there is another child or grownup to play with.

But Emma has to deal with contradictory feelings just as I do. "I wish I had a plain brother," she says one day. My heart skips a beat. I take a deep breath and ask her what a plain brother would be like. "He would walk and talk and he would never die," she answers promptly. I hold her and we talk about Jake. Again, I reassure her that he is doing very well now and encourage her not to worry.

In August 1997, we are at David and Hinda's new home with their children Mira and Zachary. Emma and Zachary are inseparable. They are only a week apart in age and have been playing together since their early days. Now the five-year-olds have been amusing themselves for two days non-stop and I suppose Emma is realising how different her brother is from bright Zack. It seems to evoke in her a profound sense of loss.

At bedtime that night she cries a little in my lap and says, "Mommy, I don't want Jakey to die." I rock her, nestling her head into my shoulder and tell her, "I know sweetheart. Me neither." I know we will muddle through but I wish I could make her hurt disappear and protect her from life's meaner moments.

Then, one day, Emma asks me, "Mommy, can Jake come with me to school?"

"I think so, honey. We'll just have to organize it."

"Good, because some of the kids don't believe I really have a brother."

Emma's family life is different from that of most of her friends. What is natural for her, like driving to Belleville to spend a day at Susie's Place, sometimes seems odd to the children she plays with. So the day Jake spends a morning with us at her daycare she is very proud to show her brother to her friends and answer their questions. The teachers are all very welcoming and I can tell from the sparkle in Emma's eyes that having her mom and brother at school with her friends is filling an important gap.

Sometimes I encourage her to invite a friend along on our visits to Jake's. The kids play outside in the country air and on the way home we stop for hamburgers and milkshakes and visit a mini-zoo. Sharing a fun day's outing to her brother's house with a school chum seems to help Emma integrate the disparate parts of her life.

Not long after Jake visits the daycare, one of Emma's favourite teachers tells me that when the kids go for a walk, she sometimes points out where Jake's tree is planted. She tells the teacher that when she and her mommy miss him, we go and see his tree by the water and say, "Hi Jake across the lake." It's good to hear this from a sympathetic teacher, a reassuring validation of the ways I've devised to help Emma feel that her brother is part of our family. And I am glad she feels comfortable enough to share this part of her life with her friends and significant grownups.

That summer when she is five and Jake is seven, he is again struck by a virus. Emma and I are in Belleville and while she pulls out toys in the playroom, I hold Jake. With his body folded like a pretzel in my lap, he looks at me and I realize how little ready I am to let him go. After all these years of holding on, I simply don't know how.

I rub his willowy back and my hand flinches away from his hot flesh. With a damp white cloth, I try to soothe the burning of his fever. His body is still, as if he is suspended in time while the medicine wrestles down the intruding infection. I cover his face, try to kindle a round of peekaboo, but his eyes, tired and hollow, are listless.

"What will it be like when Jakey dies?" Emma asks me later in the car. As always, I tell her that he will go gently, in peace, and that she should not worry. When she asks me again, only a few days later, I am aware that her burden is not lightened by my response. In reality, I do not have an answer to her question, her anguish and longing for understanding beyond her years. Death remains a mystery to us both.

Jake is paper-thin, his skin translucent, occasionally tinged with blue, especially on the tips of his slender fingers and under his expressive eyes. We take special precautions now against bed sores. He lies on foam, dimpled like an egg crate. Nothing is too good for my boy. For a second, I am reminded of the *Princess and the Pea* and have to laugh.

Gail and I share our thoughts as usual, a checklist of good and bad signs. She fears he may experience a slow decline, his heart still strong but his other systems giving out one by one. This is not what we hope. We all want a quick and painless death for him, for ourselves. We cluck our worry, taking comfort in the familiarity now, after almost seven years of the roller coaster ride together. We tease one another that Jake keeps us on our toes, bouncing back from death's door to greet us, smiling, again.

It is morning and I hear Jake's cough greeting the sunlight as it enters his room. From the doorway I see droplets of sweat on his forehead, testimony to the fire that burns inside while he sleeps. For me, it is a day like others, of passing time trying to drink Jakey up, cherishing the moments together. Sometimes I am able to keep my fear at bay, to focus squarely on the moments at hand. I have heard it said that God has lent us our children. This begins to have meaning for me as we linger together.

I love him. Every nook and cranny of his slight body. His wheezing breath and arms and legs, flailing higgledy-piggledy while he sits in his chair. He takes in his surroundings, always with a wise, almost knowing look. We will never know how much he sees, what he can process in his brain that stopped growing so soon after his beginning.

And yet, during the last couple of months, we have all noticed signs of cognitive development. How can it be? Even while his systems march resolutely toward shutdown, he reaches for a toy, on purpose, after it has been removed from his grasp.

If I let myself, I can become quite morose at the prospect of facing a day without him. He has given me purpose, passion. His smile lights up my heart and even the word *love* has new meaning: a tolerant, observant caring that asks little in return. It is morning and we will face the day together.

Emma's second birthday coincided with one of Jake's brushes with death. Now she is to turn six in a couple of weeks and says, "I want Jakey to come to my birthday party."

"That's a nice idea, honey," I say, trying to work out the logistics in my mind. Her party this year is at a bowling alley and I'm not sure how we'll get Jake there and take care of him while twelve other children are bowling. "I'll talk to Daddy about it, okay?"

Jim and I decide it is too hard to coordinate everyone's activities, do the preparation for the party and go to pick up Jake from Belleville; the volunteer driving service was discontinued several years ago. It's too bad, because it is lovely that Emma wants to include her brother. I tell her that we'll have a special birthday party for her at Susie's Place soon after her regular party. The prospect of more than one birthday celebration does wonders.

"You hate me," Emma tells me one morning with all the venom her little being can muster. We are at odds because I want her to get dressed for school. I have raised my voice and she does not like it.

"Well, I certainly don't hate you," I tell her.

"Well, you never yell at Jakey," she says.

"But I get mad at him sometimes too. You just don't see me."

"When?" she asks.

"Sometimes when he's sick," I answer.

"But he can't help it," she says, protective of her brother. This kind of conversation is becoming more common between us as Emma sorts out how her brother is different. She is realizing that he has special needs, although she doesn't put it that way. She is also very sure that he has the same rights as all other kids.

Her rights seem to include taking forever to get dressed and out the door. I am reminded of the political slogan "The struggle continues," an apt title for a video about mornings in our house. This strategic thinking has taken on a whole new focus.

Shortly before she starts grade one, Emma and I visit Jake. He's in pretty good shape, his breathing relatively clear. He is amazingly responsive to sound and touch, even to sight. He smiles readily and chuckles. As I take him into the washroom to change his diaper, he anticipates the light game. He grins knowingly as I turn the light on the first time. I sit him upright, leaning him back against the warmth of my chest so he faces the large mirror. Emma and I make faces at him, turning the light on and off. He smiles when the light lingers on his handsome face. He is a big boy now, tall, and his constant wriggling makes him a challenge to hold comfortably.

Though he is doing well just now, at times he needs to be watched carefully for suctioning. It is wonderful to watch him and Emma together. She helps me suction him when he needs it; she is growing into such a mature, caring little girl.

"That boy has problems, like Jake," she tells me, indicating a young boy we can see through the window. We are sitting on stools at a cafe near her school late one afternoon. This is Emma's favourite spot for a treat with her mom or dad or any other adult who offers. "He has problems, like my brother," she tells me, proud to have made such an observation. "I wonder where he lives."

I am aware that she is constantly processing this kind of information, wondering how and where kids like her brother live. She is not afraid to talk about Jake. Quite the contrary, she always describes her family as including him. And now she will speak about his death freely. She tells me that it's a good thing I have her, so I won't always be sad, like if I lost two children. "What would you do if I was like Jake?" she asks me one morning.

"I'd love you an awful lot," I said.

"But what if we both died and you were alone?"

"I think I'd be sad for many days," I answered.

She plays out these little scenarios, as if to try them on for size. I hope her ability to verbalize this worry will ease her brother's actual passing.

It is not as easy to make special occasions of Jake's birthdays as it is for Emma but in May 1995 he is five years old, a huge milestone for all of us. A vivid picture fills my mind: of a happy boy, giving me a squeeze and running eagerly into his kindergarten class. It is not meant to be. Still, we will celebrate the fullness of these five years in our own way.

And so I plan a ritual to mark Jake's entry into our community, his coming of age. It seems strange at first but, as I read and talk with

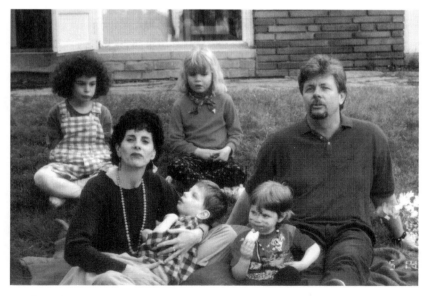

Family and guests at Jake's Bar Mitzvah, 1995.

the women in my Jewish studies group, my thoughts come together. Jake may not live to be thirteen so it feels right to make him a Bar Mitzvah now. I spend days and nights reading about Jewish rituals and their meaning, trying out different ideas on Jim, who is marvellously open to this adventure. I so much appreciate this about him; I am given room to develop in ways I find valuable. He doesn't share my commitment to Jewish study or practice but still supports what I propose for our family. I evolve a service to be held outside in our backyard, under the trees.

The morning is hazy, threatening rain but the moment we begin the service, the clouds part. It is a perfect day. Fifty or sixty friends and our families, some who have traveled long distances to be with us, gather in the backyard which overlooks Lake Ontario. Jim and I thank our friends for their love and support.

We speak of *Tikkun Olam*, Hebrew words meaning "to heal, repair and transform the world" through our actions together.

We speak of Elijah the prophet, the guardian of children, and how when the Messiah comes, children like Jake will not have to struggle for what they need—not only to survive, but to live well.

We speak of learning to live life fully in the knowledge of Jake's early death, to face and cherish this most painful contradiction for a parent. We acknowledge the challenge, from Jake's very first breath, of not having an accurate road map, of never knowing what to expect for him.

Together we sing *Hinea Ma Tov*, from Psalm 133, which means, "Behold, how good and how pleasant it is when brothers and sisters dwell together in unity."

We tell our friends that Emma-Maryse is going to plant a tree for her brother later this week in the Gatineau Hills. In Judaism, the cedar symbolizes strength and stature. (We won't discuss the fact that for girls, one is meant to plant a cypress sapling, which symbolizes gentleness and sweetness.)

Many of us read favourite passages, talk about Jake and remember all we have to be thankful for. Some of the children read poems they have written.

After the service, my father-in-law thanks me for letting him say goodbye to his grandson in a joyful way. A friend tells us that much of what we shared would usually have gone unsaid until the person's death.

For me too, there is finally some closure. We have managed to inject a tiny bit of control into this otherwise random journey that is Jake's life. We have created a vibrant and positive milestone that endures for us and will last well beyond his presence with us.

And that, in a nutshell, is Jake's gift. His stay with us is temporary, as we have known for most of his life, but the meaning of his life endures and continues to enrich our days. Being Jake's parent has caused me to reinvent myself in ways I could never have imagined.

I have always tried to nurture a line of communication between Emma and her brother. Playful fantasies like the treats he hides for her, the songs we sing with messages to each other, are all part of this effort.

One night, just after Emma's seventh birthday, we are visiting with my parents at their apartment. During dinner she describes our last visit to Jakey's. She tells her grandparents that *she* can understand what her brother is trying to say. "Brothers and sisters have a special language, you know."

11

Families Fight Back

I T IS A COLD NIGHT in January 1995. Outside, a snow squall threatens to wrestle traffic to a crawl. Where I am sitting, it is dry and warm. I'm in a large meeting room packed with women and men speaking in Italian, Polish and Punjabi. Each has just received a letter that says the Thistletown Regional Treatment Centre, where we are now gathered, is to close in six months. Feelings run high, even before the meeting is called to order. Thistletown is their anchor, the provider of specialized and innovative programs that help their kids. This otherwise diverse group is linked by the presence in their lives of children who, like my four-and-a-half-year-old Jake, grapple with severe emotional, developmental and behavioural challenges. For the parents of Thistletown children, closing the facility would spell disaster. Their lives are already more chaotic than usual. They are struggling to hold down jobs, raise their families and provide for their loved ones who happen to have special needs. For any family, it's a huge set of demands.

The Thistletown Centre is often referred to as the last stop for troubled kids. It opened as a children's mental health and research facility in 1958 and is now the largest professional training centre in Canada in its field. The Centre functions in co-operation with the community, as schools and recreation facilities are utilized for many of its activities, which serve more than four hundred families in five specialized programs. It employs three hundred people in a variety of professional capacities, offering some residential care—between ten and fifteen treatment beds.

One program treats teenagers whose behaviour points to learning disabilities or psychiatric challenges. These conduct disorders, as they are called, can be complex and confounding. Thistletown helps improve care by sharing information between psychiatrists working in this field.

Another program provides a unique opportunity to children who are sexually abused, and their families. Treatment features a holistic approach; specialists are involved in every aspect of the family's care. Issues can be explored in a comprehensive fashion, a method that has earned the program an international reputation in curbing sexual abuse. As with its other programs, where clinical practice is honed over years of experience, Thistletown provides training to university faculty and other professionals.

Children living with autism and other developmental challenges receive multi-disciplinary care in partnership with community schools. Thistletown provides last resort residential care for a small number of young people, as well as vitally important parent-relief programs. Special education teachers work with each child on an individualized program. Sometimes kids spend weekends on site to allow family members to catch their breath. Reliable transportation to and from services is available for children. Finally, integrated research allows the Centre to develop a database unmatched in Canada.

Troubled families may also be helped to stay together, instead of having to resort to residential care. Thistletown staff work in concert with the Children's Aid Society to offer intensive family therapy, special classroom supports, and home support services. More than two hundred families receive assistance through this program each year.

Thistletown staff care for troubled and seriously ill children and youth. Frequently clients and their families are frighteningly close to coming unhinged. By providing expertise and resources in a controlled environment, including recreation facilities, an extensive library, and audio-visual materials, significant advances are achieved. Information about successes, as well as setbacks, is shared with other agencies through staff development opportunities, and by collaborating on clinical programming.

At the front of the meeting room, a woman I later get to know as Sandra Bradley invites everyone to pick up copies of official-looking documents from the table beside her. She knows several of the participants by name. When the formal part of the meeting begins, she makes a few comments about the government's announcement and then throws the floor open for comments.

For about an hour, parents describe all the ways in which services offered by Thistletown have made life possible, often much better, for them and their families. They tell stories with varying degrees of reserve; not everyone wants to bare her soul, but it is clear that a sense of purpose is developing.

Sandra and Richard Bradley's son Nathan attends a special day program designed for kids with autism. When he was seventeen or eighteen months old, his parents noticed something was not quite right. He barely slept and tended to "climb the walls." He seemed unaware of others in his environment. His parents thought he might be deaf and took him to an early intervention response team. By the time Nathan was almost two and a half, they got the diagnosis: Nathan was autistic. He would require special education and care throughout his life. He started going to Thistletown when he was four. "It was a very positive step," Richard Bradley tells the group. "It was really a question of our sanity. Nathan's attention span was measured at fifteen seconds. We had three children by that time, and the others could not compete because Nathan demanded so much. Now he is bussed to school each day. He is learning to print his name and to speak a little bit. He'll even tell you his name."

Gradually, the talk turns to action. What can the parents do to fight the government's decision to close Thistletown? Sandra encourages people to sign up for a steering committee or join groups to be responsible for public education, communications and fundraising tasks. Her capacity for organizing is obvious.

I have been invited to this meeting because I work for the Ontario Public Service Employees Union, OPSEU, but as the parent of a special needs child, I sympathize as deeply with the parents' needs as with the employees'. I'm sitting beside Michael Stohr, president of OPSEU Local 547 at Thistletown, who phoned me when rumours of impending layoffs reached him. He offers families the staff's support; his members—social workers, physical and psychological therapists of all descriptions, kitchen workers and administrative staff—provide care to Thistletown's kids and young people. Tonight Thistletown staff is working for free to babysit the children, including siblings, so that parents can meet together without interruption.

Michael and I met for the first time earlier this evening, just outside the building. News of the closure had already hit the press and the staff was concerned; they knew that layoff notices would soon follow. We hit it off immediately, largely because we shared a similar outlook on community organizing. We did not require a major discussion of first principles in order to build resistance to an unjust situation. We had agreed over the telephone that we needed to hear the parents' views on the closure and offer them the union's full support to fight it. He cautioned that management might not allow us into the meeting that evening. I suggested we try anyway, since it was a meeting called by parents, not the employer, and it was their decision to include or exclude the union from discussions. In my view, we had nothing to lose by showing up at the appointed time.

To the surprise of neither of us, the Centre's administrator tried to detour us just as we entered the meeting room. She indicated that the gathering was for parents only. I puffed up to my full five-foot-four-inch stature and assured her that we were simply there to offer the union's assistance. We would not lead or take over, but support whatever course of action the families settled upon.

Since I am not an employee, I have no reason to fear any sanction. At the worst, we would have waited around outside and spoken informally with the parents as they left the grounds. If I have learned anything from working with the CAW boys, it is that you can talk yourself into most any gathering with the right combination of firmness and diplomacy. Above all, you need a sense of humour. It can be the most disarming tool in the shit-disturber's arsenal. While the administrator looked at us somewhat quizzically, we slipped in.

We are sitting at the back of the room. Michael greets some of the parents by name. It is obvious that the link between a youth worker like Michael and these families is important—not unlike the one I experience when I pick up my daughter from her daycare in the afternoon. Information is shared about highlights of the day and progress made in significant areas. We are all participants in the raising of our children and, when it works, the relationship is friendly and supportive. I know the value of Michael's rapport with the parents of these special needs' families.

The task tonight is to build on the trust between families and the Centre's staff and its union. While our members watch over their charges next door at the pool and gymnasium, a photographer takes pictures of the kids at play. It will take a significant head of steam to stem the government's decision; photographs or film can better portray the special quality of expertise and service OPSEU members offer these vulnerable young people.

At the end of the meeting, Michael and I stay on to chat with the steering committee volunteers. We introduce ourselves to the parents who shared their stories and make sure they know where to reach us. Michael again pledges the Thistletown staff's support. We offer meeting space at our office and to type and photocopy any materials they need. Michael adds that the union local will activate its steward network to help distribute information to each family.

I explain that my area of expertise is government lobbying and media relations. I also mention that I have a child who requires special care. When they ask about Jake's situation, I give them copies of a couple of articles I have written about fighting for Jake's care. That's when the walls come tumbling down. We are part of the same club—fighting for our kids' right to services is a way of life. Michael and I are invited to join the parents when their committee meets later that week.

For the staff, the closure would mean redeployment if they are lucky and losing their jobs if not. Almost every social agency is in cutback mode due to federal and provincial funding constraints. Although waiting lists for services are not diminishing, jobs in the social service sector are in jeopardy. In the union's estimation, closing Thistletown is a bad precedent for other beleaguered mental health facilities in the province.

The Centre's programs cost taxpayers several million dollars a year. The provincial government plans to transfer $12.2 million into what it calls "community-based" services. Public and private agencies, many of which have been starved for adequate financing, are clamouring for this money. The government claims further that about $2 million will be saved in administrative costs and salaries. Meanwhile, waiting lists for a range of children's services including speech therapy, behaviour modification, crisis intervention and family counselling are getting longer. Thistletown's programs and expertise cannot be provided by a mishmash of agencies and workers making home visits.

The government, however, has gravely misjudged the community's reaction. From that first night in January the Thistletown parents, with OPSEU's support, mount a fierce campaign. After a meeting or two, they decide to call themselves FFACT: Families and Friends Against Closing Thistletown.

With superb energy and creativity, Sandra sets to producing buttons and designing letterhead. She phones the Ministry of Community and Social Services almost daily, demanding to speak with the Ministry's point man for the closure project. Richard paints "Save Thistletown" on his van. He often travels around town with young Nathan on his shoulders. A computer expert with a talent for communications, he programs his home fax machine to broadcast information to the steering committee and the Toronto media. Several other parents play key roles in our community outreach, winning support from their faith groups, school boards, unions, teachers and local merchants. Every person has a skill to share.

I contribute lobbying strategy, news releases, intensive schmoozing of the press and preparing OPSEU officials for high level meetings with the ministry. We examine the Minister's and the Premier's messages to the press and public to decipher the meaning behind the bland statements. As in hard bargaining with any opponent, we watch for signals. This helps me to know where pressure needs to be applied—the Ministry of Community and Social Services, the New Democratic Party caucus or the Premier's office, for example. By pinpointing the levers of power we can best access, we marshal our energy and resources effectively.

We employ similar strategic thinking to our relations with the public, through the media. At best, media relations are a two-way street. We share and receive vital information through these exchanges as the press also speaks directly with government and agency officials. A few journalists cover the story with great assiduity as it unfolds. Several OPSEU staff colleagues help to organize outreach in the community and to evaluate members' options should layoff notices be issued in April, as announced. For the union, it is crucial that we address our members' bread and butter concerns regarding their livelihoods in addition to fighting the social and political battle to preserve services essential to the community.

The parents run the show, with a strong union presence in the background. Michael and I manage, stone by stone, to build the level of trust this kind of community organizing requires. Getting along is something people in coalitions generally have to work at and we know that parents and the union have separate interests that happen to come together toward a common goal, keeping the Centre open.

When Minister Tony Silipo tries (unsuccessfully) to placate the parents and staff at an evening meeting near Thistletown, we are there. TV news that night shows over two hundred people doing the wave with a simple bright yellow photocopied sheet that says "Save Thistletown." OPSEU president Fred Upshaw is at the meeting but declines to take the podium saying, "This is the families' meeting. We are here to support them, not steal the show."

On certain questions, the union and parents' steering committee have to agree to disagree but on the central questions, we are able to maintain unity. The parents understand clearly that the workers they see each day, the people who are committed to their children, are also union members with families and responsibilities of their own. They understand that if these people lose their jobs, the quality of care their children receive will be compromised. The bonds forged through this common interest and our activities and lively discussions are strong.

In late February 1995, the government announces that it will delay issuing layoff notices. Our members and FFACT know this to be a turning point. Certainly we claim it as a mini-victory in the larger battle. No question, the government's change of heart is due, in part, to the parents' and union's delivery of a consistent message. When the media push the families, the parents again say, "No layoffs."

We have only won a delay and we continue our strategy: to create a ruckus and use every ally we can identify. This means school boards, health boards and municipal councils. Some of the Thistletown parents are involved on the municipal scene in their communities. They make sure the closure issue is raised in a variety of public forums with their neighbours and local newspapers.

For OPSEU, this outreach is a necessary prelude to "getting a table," that is, to opening discussions where the employment issues will be negotiated with the government. We ask to meet with representatives for the Ministry of Community and Social Services. No doubt, their spin doctors are working overtime too.

Throughout, I encourage the FFACT steering committee members to take turns handling the daily media interviews that our activities (and systematic phone calls) are drumming up: "no stars allowed" is a good rule of thumb. As the campaign gains force, influential columnists meet with us. Editorials appear in key newspapers; radio and television interviews are seen and heard frequently. Wherever possible, the children and families are shown in their homes to give an idea of the texture of their lives. The campaign is building into a classic David and Goliath battle where disadvantaged children and youth are pitted against the powers of government and those who want to slash social service budgets.

We organize noisy demonstrations and public meetings and sometimes some of the Thistletown children come along with staff by their side, attending to their needs. Emma often joins us. Teams of union members and parents set up information pickets. The children's vulnerability is illustrated graphically in community newspapers and television news items. We are able to show the public that most of Thistletown's care is delivered in the community, not in the institution.

Support rolls in from major unions, teachers, school boards and medical professionals. Some senior specialists write letters to the papers on our behalf. One, referring to the clinical research and treatment record of the Thistletown Centre, says, "No one else offers the depth of programming and treatment. . . . There are so many boutiques out there; sometimes you need a general store. If you lose those connections you lose the depth to experiment with new ideas and treatments."

Many mornings, Sandra and I speak on the phone before our kids are awake. We evaluate the previous day and check details for the hours ahead. I attempt to provide her and the other FFACT members with personal encouragement, as well as technical support. It is a hectic time and these families still have to manage the rest of their lives.

Parents and union members write letters and make numerous presentations to school boards, municipal councils and health boards. These bodies pass motions against the closure and write to the Minister for Community and Social Services. Some of the parents, their kids and staff do interviews with the press almost daily. Together we are building up pressure that the government cannot afford to ignore.

Fairly early on, Minister Silipo indicates publicly to the families that if adequate services did not exist in the community, the Centre would not close. I believe this statement to be significant; it opens an important window. If we can demonstrate that the services are not available, then the parents and staff will maintain the moral high ground. Clearly, the focus of our efforts has to be to illustrate the glaring gap in community services, contrary to defensive government messages. Consequently we pull out all stops with the public outreach and media relations strategy. Each day, another municipality or school board declares its support for FFACT's position and *The Toronto Star* runs more than one lead editorial condemning the government's decision to close Thistletown.

The media are alert to such stories. Only a few months before, a tragic murder-suicide attracted considerable attention. A mother killed herself and her sixteen-year-old disabled son. It was gruesome. And coverage of the death of twelve-year-old Tracey Latimer in Saskatchewan in 1994 led to heightened awareness of the challenges facing children with special needs. In my daily exchanges with the press during the Thistletown campaign, the lesson of this harrowing tragedy is never far from the surface.

Inside OPSEU, I argue that we need to initiate a broad public debate about the issues raised in the policy tradeoffs between residential care and people's right to live in the community. There is a strong popular opinion that residential care for all people with disabilities is outdated. This well-meaning view has given the opponents of good social services an excuse to reduce overall expenditure on care. I do not believe, however, that funding grabbed from residential care is going to find its way into appropriate community services.

For the disability movement, self-determination and greater individual control for people receiving public services are vital, foundational tenets. They include independence of movement and greater access. In the past, the rights of those who need services have been disgracefully ignored but the solution, surely, is not to dismantle but to improve such services.

OPSEU members are often the ones who provide public services as employees of the state. It is their job to enforce the rules that regulate the programs they deliver, rules they have not made but which are established elsewhere, by statute or policy of the governing party. And sometimes, these rules go against the express wishes of people on the receiving end of services. Our members understand that care recipients and families are fed up with the runaround they often receive from various agencies and public bodies. No one is well-served by a system rife with outrageous waiting lists and understaffing. Union members working in this field endorse policy and practice that treats people with disabilities with dignity—even if the resources assigned by government are inadequate.

The staff at Thistletown understand the value of a centre that provides care both in the community and in a residential setting. Further, they know from professional experience that individual needs change over time. A person who, at one time, is able to live well in the community with appropriate supports may, at another time, require residential care. And if the family's needs change, due perhaps to a mother's illness or death, they may have to call more heavily on Thistletown programs to remain intact. As the Child and Family Service Act states, children's services should be provided in a manner that "respects children's needs to continuity of care and for stable family relationships." That's precisely what Thistletown has come to mean to both its clients and staff.

Nathan Bradley, for example, spends several weekends each season at the parent relief program at Thistletown. "It allows us to do some of the family activities we need to, especially for the other kids," says Richard. "It is the only way."

Residential care and increased service options in the community are not mutually exclusive options. During the campaign we attempt to correct the mistaken impression that Thistletown operated at arm's-length from the community and to show that many of its programs are being delivered at sites such as schools and recreation facilities in communities where clients live.

While employment issues such as wages, benefits, job security and adequate training opportunities are central, the union also has a commitment to quality public services. Families should be able to make informed choices about the kind of care that suits their particular needs; the system should be set up to provide for this.

The union advocates a broad range of supports, including residential care and respite care, sibling and parent counselling as well as a vast array of essential therapies. At the same time, it is our belief that all privately-employed caregivers should receive a decent salary and benefits for their skilled, dedicated work, on a par with their unionized colleagues. However, for governments, private entrepreneurship in the health and disability sectors means cutting costs by eroding wages.

The need for different advocacy groups to work together for resources is illustrated when the Ontario government is getting pilloried in the press for closing Thistletown. They announce an infusion of cash to the Special Services at Home (SSAH) program. It funds certain elements of care for children with disabilities who live at home. The amount is a drop in the bucket, according to an advocacy group representing these parents, but the announcement's timing was surely more than coincidence. Some of the Thistletown parents are furious.

It is important to make it known that the government's announcement is meant to take the wind out of FFACT's sails, to pit them against other groups in the community. In fact, both kinds of funding are required—our kids have a range of needs. Some months earlier, a colleague and I hosted a meeting with the families receiving SSAH and it had become clear that we did not share the same approach to labour relations issues, particularly with respect to employment rights under the government's individualized funding model.

On the day the government's funding announcement is to be made, Sandra Bradley and a couple of other FFACT members join me at the legislature media studio. The union's government liaison officer has received word of the announcement and a couple of reporters I work closely with have advised me of the afternoon conference. We listen to the press conference and I tell the media that our representative is also prepared to comment.

We make it clear that we will not allow the ministry to pit parent against parent. Both kinds of programs for kids with disabilities are necessary—and starved for funds. The Thistletown parents express their support for the SSAH parents' group, although they fear the announcement signals a further rejection of the coordinated care offered at Thistletown.

The ability to rise above one's particular issue is not inbred. When the proverbial pie is getting smaller, people naturally fear they will be deprived of their slice. But we know that if we work together where possible and remain focused on achieving better funding for all children with disabilities, much can be achieved. The needs of these two sets of families are not that different. Although the government services they make use of are organized under separate models, they face the same barriers to involvement in the workforce.

A recent study found that 39 percent of the sample reported their employment status had been affected by their responsibilities as parents of children with special needs. And fully 64 percent of two-parent families with one parent unemployed reported their child's special needs were a major factor in the parent being at home. Like all parents, the lack of access to appropriate, affordable licensed childcare was a significant barrier to their own ability to work outside the home. Correspondingly, 88 percent of these parents reported being tired and overloaded and 90 percent said they were stressed about balancing work and family obligations.

It's more than likely that the families active in FFACT experience similar rates of stress. As well as the best possible care for their kids, they required greater flexibility in their shift schedules and in making use of leave provisions to meet their children's care requirements. Frequent medical appointments, illnesses, and added expenses due to the equipment and medications their kids require are also common concerns which fuelled their determination to keep Thistletown open.

In late March, we participate in a large public debate on the future of the Greater Toronto Area. *The Toronto Star* is sponsoring the event held at the plush Royal York Hotel. My colleagues and I decide it is time to unveil our secret weapon—a new superhero to be known as the Defender of Public Services. At lunch that day, I zoom off to a store to look over the costumes available. I settle on a red, blue, and white Superwoman outfit.

On the way back to the office I drop the costume at Richard and Sandra's. She is an accomplished seamstress, in addition to caring for three children, fundraising and having more energy than any one person should be allowed. By suppertime, our superhero's royal blue cape sports large red letters proclaiming "Public Defender: Services For People."

Several of us fly (figuratively) down to the hotel in Richard's van with its Save Thistletown signs. We set up on the sidewalk as crowds began to file in the hotel entrance. Distributing flyers, waving picket signs and speaking with passersby keeps us busy until show time. I have the honour of playing the hero, wearing sharp-looking red boots over white tights, flinging my colourful cape into the wind.

It's time to go in and we are warned that no costumes or picket signs are allowed. We leave the picket signs outside and someone drapes a coat over my shoulders. About ten of us file in, including Richard with young Nathan sitting on his shoulders.

After the opening speeches, people line up at the microphones. One of the Thistletown staff and I stand at a mike waiting our turn. Of course I take the opportunity to disrobe, revealing the Super-woman costume and slogan, before asking a question about Thistle-town. The photographers and television cameras have a field day. It's too late and too amusing for the authorities to give us the boot. Once again, we make the news, keeping Thistletown's future squarely on the public agenda.

By mid-April the government has had enough of our shenanigans. Besides, it is increasingly evident that they have made a poor decision. They need a way out. After a few more demonstrations and high-level meetings at the ministry, Minister Silipo says he has heard the concerns of the families and "it is very clear to (him) that there has been a breakdown in trust." He announces a moratorium on the closure, pending an independent review.

The mutually respectful relationship between parents and staff has been central to the campaign's success, building up trust, allowing space for one another's separate interests, and then co-operating where possible. No doubt the experience staff and parents already have had in working together on behalf of their children in the therapeutic setting has helped a lot.

For OPSEU, it has meant making a strategic decision to put public service issues at the forefront. The union did not highlight the issue of jobs. Instead, we pushed for maintaining the programs that families relied upon. But when the government started threatening to move the staff out, the parents spoke out vociferously about the need to maintain continuity of care for their children. It was the parents who fought for our members' jobs.

The Thistletown organizing was a success because we valued the experience, skills, and sense of humour that individuals brought with them. Creativity and fun were part of keeping people engaged in the effort.

For me personally, it was a wonderful opportunity to connect with families not unlike my own and to be reminded, again, how Jake's life has fuelled my passion to engage in these activities. He gives me a remarkable sense of purpose and focus in my social and political interventions, as a citizen and a mom.

For Nathan Bradley, as for many Thistletown kids, his parents' determination carried the day. "The campaign was utter chaos," Richard says in retrospect. "But we were successful and that's what counts." After years of fighting on behalf of their children for the right to access health and community services, the Thistletown parents are not going to budge. This quality, together with their absolute refusal to accept defeat, has made their resistance a success. Later in April 1995, the government confirms the moratorium, pending an independent review of the families' needs and what community agencies could realistically provide. A report is issued later that year, and by the end of 1999 the Mike Harris Conservative Government has still chosen not to reopen this Pandora's box. If it does, parents, caregivers and their union will be there to stop them. Nathan and all the other children deserve the best shot at life we can give them.

12

The Ethic of Care

SIX MONTHS after the decision to keep Thistletown open, we have another battle to fight. It's November of 1995; Jake is feeling reasonably well and it's time to sign his one-year renewal agreement for care at Susie's Place. Each year since 1990, the signing of the Special Needs Agreement has been quite routine. We meet with the CAS social worker and Gail to discuss Jake's health. Sometimes it's emotional but not controversial. Jake needs care; Susie's Place provides it. The CAS funnels money (our tax dollars) from the Ministry of Community and Social Services in the form of a per diem (which varies from $160 to $300) and the Ministry of Health funds certain equipment and medications. We are fortunate that our health insurance plans from work pick up the rest.

But this year, a change of government in Ontario means the CAS budget is squeezed to the max. The agency threatens to send Jake home unless we pay a substantial monthly user's fee. When this issue was raised the previous year, we resisted. We didn't have the money, but it was also an ideological question. Canadian health care services are not meant to carry user fees. We won our point, but this year, the agency officials are playing hardball. Jake will be moved out of a facility paid for via the CAS and sent either to another agency

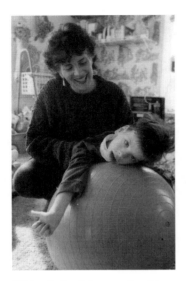

Miriam helps Jake stretch at his group home.

paid for directly by the province (like a hospital) or be sent home.

Jim and I are appalled. The reasoning is faulty. Jake needs the sophisticated level of care that Susie's Place provides. Home is not an option, nor will I let him live in hospital or a facility of any lesser quality. Besides, the eventual source of funding is the same, the Ontario taxpayers, and a hospital bed would cost them a great deal more. It would be absurd to move him when he is responding well and we have all worked so hard (especially Gail and myself) to develop a co-operative team approach to raising him.

Anger does not begin to describe my reaction. We feel robbed of control over our lives. Here is Jake, never more than a virus away from dire consequences, and budget cuts are calling the shots. It's simply not acceptable.

Jim and I decide to fight back. Once again, I rally all of my advocacy skills, this time in Jake's (and our) defense. Never is it harder to advocate for justice, it seems, than for oneself.

I contact a *Toronto Star* reporter who meets Jim and me to nail down the details of our story. Late that night, I drive out to Belleville so a photographer can do a midnight photo shoot with Jake and me at the group home. I know from my work in media relations that a photo will help drive the story.

I also call our member of the provincial legislature. Caucus research staff gather pertinent facts to broaden the story and give it context. In the days that follow, a photo of Jake and me appears on the front page of *The Toronto Star*, the newspaper with the highest circulation in the country. That afternoon, Bob Rae, leader of the New Democratic Party, is to ask a question in the House about Jake's plight and that of families like ours.

I assemble a group of parents and children with disabilities to accompany me to the legislature and we sit in the visitors' gallery overlooking the politicians' benches. A parent from the Safehaven Association for Community Living is with us and at my side is my friend from the Thistletown battle, Sandra Bradley.

I have warned Sandra, gently, that we have to respect the decorum of the House. The stately atmosphere, paintings, and ornate ceilings heighten the formality of the proceedings below. Jim sits on my other side and squeezes my hand as we listen to the debate.

Bob Rae asks his question about Jake, referring to the article in the morning's paper. Conservative Cabinet Minister Dave Tsubouchi (the bright light who recommended poor people negotiate with grocery clerks for cheaper cans of tuna) tries to skate around the issue. Mr. Rae poses supplementary questions, waving Jake's picture emphatically at the government benches. The third time Mr. Tsubouchi waffles and weaves, I just lose it.

"You're going to kill my child," I scream, standing up in horror.

Instantly, a rather large gentleman pushes past Jim to silence me. My husband stands six foot one and weighs enough to qualify for work as a bouncer, but the gendarme will have none of Jim's explanations. We are swiftly thrown out of the Legislature.

The guard leads me, shaking, down the steps from the gallery and away from television cameras. We gather outside the visitors' gallery around the water cooler and take a few deep breaths. I am just beginning to regain my composure when Sandra jostles me.

"Oh yeah, Miriam, and you told *me* to behave!"

Our ejection from the Legislature brings more media attention to the issue of funding care for medically-fragile children. Another article and photo of Jake appear in *The Toronto Star*; *The Globe and Mail*, *The Ottawa Citizen* and other newspapers also carry the story.

One of the most bizarre elements of this episode is the reaction of a newly-elected Conservative backbencher, John Baird. (At the end of 1999 he is Minister of Community and Social Services.) We had recently faced off in a TV debate about the consequences of his government's program for working people. Today, he responds to my outburst by yelling, "She's an OPSEU member."

Hansard, as well as news stories the next day, show that one of Mr. Baird's fellow members urged him to pipe down. He didn't, much to his chagrin, I suspect. Articles and newspaper columns appear later that week suggesting his comments were ill-advised and people send unsolicited letters of protest to the government and the newspapers. We hear that some elementary school teachers have made bulletin board displays based on this incident and encouraged children to write advocacy letters on Jake's behalf.

This experience is both exciting and exhausting—my instincts as a professional communications specialist have worked nicely. But genuine passion and concern propelled me. I simply seized the moment.

In the fall of 1996, Laura Sky's video *Jake's Life* is screened and a TV current affairs program does a piece about Jake and our struggles as a family. They show clips from the film, interspersed with an interview with me about advocating for children's rights. Laura and her crew shot the film in 1995, starting with Jake's Bar Mitzvah celebration. It tells the story of his struggles for health and how we fought to preserve his care at Susie's Place.*

To my surprise, the TV interviewer asks me to comment on the episode at the Legislature earlier that year. She wants to know what compelled me to go public with Jake's story.

"What choice did we have?" I respond. For me, and for other parents I have encountered in this movement, the answer is simple: our kids cannot speak for themselves.

As a result of this advocacy Jake's funding was reinstated some months later, no further questions asked. I subsequently received a supportive letter from Mr. Bruce Rivers, the executive director of the Toronto Children's Aid Society, congratulating me for being a "passionate spokesperson for these children who cannot speak for themselves."

All parents have battles to fight for their children's care. We must be ready to go public and make noise. For Jim and me, this fight comes

---

* The thirty-two-minute video *Jake's Life* is available from SkyWorks at (416) 536- 6581.

naturally. We demonstrate and raise hell for a living. Others may have to reach deep inside themselves to find the strength to make such a ruckus. Even for us, however, it is a profoundly disturbing and difficult time. I grapple with an uncomfortable level of anxiety for months; worrying whether your child will have appropriate care is very draining. I have to take steps to avoid becoming completely strung out.

I will never forgive the powers that be for, in effect, stealing away those months of Jake's life from us. Instead of spending Saturday afternoons cuddling little Jake in my arms or taking Emma out for a toboggan ride, I have been writing letters to the editor and crafting opinion pieces for newspapers and radio stations.

Fortunately, true to form, our friends and union sisters and brothers recognize the high stakes of the battle and offer us a great deal of emotional support. Unlike many parents in our situation we are not left alone, accompanied only by feelings of impotence or desperation.

Since I first read about Saskatchewan farmer Robert Latimer, who killed his twelve-year-old daughter Tracy because he believed her suffering was unbearable, I have been struck by the parallels with Jake. There is a look in both children's eyes, likely brought on by the potent medications their conditions dictate. I have felt compelled to examine my own views about mercy killing. In August 1995, Mr. Latimer was criticized harshly on moral grounds. I write to the *Globe and Mail*:

> As a parent of a profoundly disabled child, who is as ill as Tracy Latimer was before her death, I must respond to the concerns raised in letters to the editor by some members of the disabled community that a more lenient judgment of mercy-killing could turn into "open season" on the disabled.
>
> I understand the fear that is being expressed. We know just how awfully human beings can treat one another in the guise of all sorts of issues.
>
> But there must also be limits to the amount of pain that a person is made to endure. At present, modern science cannot always provide adequate relief from pain. What treatment does not provide, nature can. In effect, dying means the end of pain.

The fact that people cannot speak for themselves means simply that someone who cares for them is forced into the powerful role of decision-maker. Many of these individuals can still express the extent of their pain and suffering. My son, for example, does not speak, but he makes it very clear to us when he is in pain.

As such a parent, I can imagine being in Robert Latimer's shoes.

Does any person have the right to make that decision for another? I think the years of care one provides go toward earning that right. It is not necessarily the blood link of parent or sister, but the hours devoted to providing intimate care that confer that responsibility.

Are there limits? Absolutely, but the penalties must better reflect the "crime" committed. Otherwise, such caregivers will continue to be punished on the same basis as actual criminals who bear malicious intent.

The key for Robert Latimer or, God forbid, for myself, is that there is no malicious intent—that is the point of mercy-killing. Love motivates the unspeakably painful act of killing a loved one. Nothing more, nothing less. And our legal system ought to be in a position to govern accordingly.

In November 1997 the news is disheartening. Latimer has been convicted of second-degree murder and awaits sentencing. The jury asked that he receive only one year's imprisonment rather than the mandatory ten years before parole is permitted. His lawyer is also planning an appeal, asking that the judge invoke a constitutional exemption that allows for leniency. It must be terrible for the Latimer family to wait, powerless, for the compassion of the court.

For me, this case is pivotal. The public debate takes on disconcerting moral overtones, a pretense, I think, that the issues are straightforward ones. Ignored is any attempt to understand the texture and quality of the lives involved.

I feel a strong empathy for Mr. Latimer and am compelled to support him and his family in this very public ordeal. The outcome of his case will touch many lives. I write an open letter to Robert Latimer and read it on CBC radio's *This Morning*. I give Mr. Latimer my best wishes and tell him,

> I truly believe you were the best father you could be. You did not deserve to be catapulted to the national screen, a monster—or hero—depending on one's perspective.
>
> In a perfect world, I point out, I suppose we humans would not be faced with such monumental ethical questions. But in the real world, the one we inhabit together, uneasily and with all our warts, your daughter's death strikes at the very core of our moral system.

All children, including Tracy Latimer, deserve to be remembered for their joyful laughter, not their screams. I say that I hope this tragedy may lead us to provide a more humane array of services for children like her and their families. A society that truly values its children would do so.

The CBC receives an enormous response; many people ask for copies of my letter, demonstrating the readiness of Canadians to engage in this debate. It is important to speak out, to expand the debate and include perspectives of those knowledgeable about disability and pain. All life deserves our fullest support but the quality of a life dominated by pain and suffering must also be considered. Tracey Latimer's death is not equivalent to the killing of a grocery store clerk. Legislation and judicial practice must include protection for those vulnerable to abuse, but not stem from a simplistic response to the situation.

For me, it has been a week of reflection and a week of action. I am reminded of our vulnerability as human beings, and that we must be prepared to speak out for justice; to ensure that lives are not wasted—or lost—due to fundamentally unfair laws.

Having a child who hovers close to death from time to time has also spurred me to look at the decision-making employed by health care practitioners. To structure my inquiry in this area, I am studying bioethics. In 1996, I attend an introductory week-long summer program at the University of Washington in Seattle. I want to know how doctors think about death and disability. What kinds of questions do they ask? How do they decide when to limit treatment?

After getting my feet wet in Seattle, I enrol in courses at the Joint Centre for Bioethics at the University of Toronto. The program brings together medical and nursing professionals with philosophers, lawyers and specialists in religious thought. Since my academic background is in the social sciences—political economy and sociology—I am not always satisfied with the tendency in the discipline to abstract bioethical issues from broader social and economic concerns. I want to cast the net wider.

Still, as in any strategic endeavour—be it social advocacy, collective bargaining, an election campaign or war—it is important to understand the logic employed by the reigning practitioners. I believe this to be critical for parents of children with disabilities, a means to adding another element to our advocacy toolbox.

Mr. Latimer is on trial while I study legal aspects of bioethics at the University of Toronto. I wonder again about the morality of his actions. If Jake were in constant pain, would I look for a similar relief to his suffering? It is hard to know. It is then that I write the "Open Letter to Robert Latimer" and read it to a national audience on radio.

Late in 1997, the OPSEU magazine, distributed to government departments, thousands of union members, and a raft of social justice organizations, features portions of that letter and a photo of Jake in an editorial highlighting the need for quality public services. Again, reaction is swift. Letters pour in, including a set of notes written by school children, their teacher having brought the issue of Mr. Latimer's sentencing forward for debate in the classroom. Another envelope arrives from an OPSEU member who teaches English as a second language to immigrants. Her class has responded to my letter, in an exercise designed to introduce them to how freedom of expression works in Canada.

In my studies, I become increasingly frustrated by the narrow purview claimed by many bioethicists. I cannot accept that decisions about life and death are made without consideration of the social and economic context. My approach is to weave together sociological inquiry with the theoretical arguments that underpin doctors' actions.

Medical schools teach doctors to preserve life. Legal practice and historical experience reinforce the imperative of life over death. Accordingly, doctors have a "duty of care" with respect to their patients. This duty permeated every aspect of my son Jake's care in the neonatal intensive care unit at the Hospital for Sick Children in Toronto in 1990. Complex care was provided him as well as detailed scientific inquiry into family history, his blood and breathing. But science could not fix Jake's condition. Mercifully he does not suffer the pain that Tracey Latimer endured but, like increasing numbers of newborns, science has saved his life but cannot equip him to live fully and independently.

My question, as a parent and informed citizen, is where the line between life and death should be drawn. And once it is established that an infant will survive for a time, where does responsibility lie for her care? My point is a practical one. We must, as a society, grapple effectively with the reality of these children's lives. With Jake's reality.

Dealing judiciously with tough issues means not flinching from talk of children's death because it is distasteful or sad. Another *duty* of care must be developed, one that corresponds to physicians' moral responsibility to keep infants alive. We have an equal responsibility to provide well for these children during their short lives, up to and including their deaths.

Law and ethics mavens are fond of bandying about different categories of justice, but often leave out the *social* justice aspect of medical decision making. Typically, questions of income, race, and power relations are considered to fall outside the formal purview of medical deliberations. But social justice theorists and feminist bioethics specialists in the United States and Canada are developing what they call the *ethic* of care.

The ethic of care arises from the notion that human interdependency is fundamental. We are persons to the extent that we relate to others. This differs sharply from the views of theorists who have for centuries defined the human self as independent, rational, self-interested, and autonomous.

While purely abstract reasoning denies the specific context of moral dilemmas, feminist bioethicists argue that moral reasoning must be rooted in specific contexts. Emotion is also recognized to play a valid role in caregiving and hence, in moral decision-making about patient care. This approach signals a sharp departure from the traditional academic view that feelings render moral decision-making impure.

What does all this mean for a child like my son? I believe that the ethic of care and notions of social justice and equity should inform social policy regarding kids like Jake. These are not just complex, airy-fairy philosophical questions to be debated in rarefied university seminars. These children require special care that our society is equipped to provide. And so we should provide it.

It is hypocritical to label as murder the failure to preserve the lives of the medically fragile, while the failure to provide care during those lives is reduced to a function of budgetary juggling.

Doctors' duty of care compels them to keep every preemie alive, with little measure of responsibility beyond the walls of the health care institution. We must, as a society, expand that duty of care throughout these children's lives—however brief. The ethic of care provides a sound basis for this shift to more comprehensive social and health policy. In the province of Ontario, it would mean changes to the Child and Family Service Act to fully mandate the extended care of medically-fragile children. There must be a commitment to help these babies live well and with dignity until they die. Nothing less is acceptable.

While most doctors probably practice non-treatment in cases where death is imminent, others are more selective and may on occasion elect not to initiate neonatal intensive care. An infant might be provided comfort care—warmth and gentle handling—and allowed to die without the administration of any painful procedures. Parents may be involved in decisions to initiate care and are always part of any decision to withdraw it.

These physicians suggest that infants and their families need protection from what one doctor calls the "caprice and tyranny of sometimes-cruel technology." The ethic of care considers the *quality* of life a value that must be balanced with a belief in the *sanctity* of life.

Of course, not all physicians or ethicists hold these opinions. Was Jake's neurologist back in 1990 justified in so adamantly refusing to discuss the quality of life our son might enjoy, with or without his G-tube? Were Jim and I meant to simply genuflect in response to expert opinion or did other options exist that could have been explored, intelligently and with compassion?

If the neurologist suspected lissencephaly soon after birth, as he suggested to us at a meeting later, why wasn't an MRI done immediately? Cost and waiting lists are no excuse. Nine years later my son is growing like a weed and there is no choice but to love and care for him. At birth, the question of his survival might have been posed and answered differently. Our family, in concert with the best medical and philosophical or spiritual advice available, should have been able to make an informed and just decision on Jake's behalf.

I accept heartily that the "default position" must be to preserve life. Certainly that is the safest route and I fully support disability activists on this point. And I reject vehemently any argument that cost of treatment determine decisions to withhold medical care. But in Jake's case, the possibility of providing comfort care alone was not open for discussion until he was six months old. I think this was wrong. Of course, determining with any accuracy which infants will survive well is a complex business. But if we possess the power, as doctors and as citizens, to keep vulnerable little ones alive then we must also exercise our judicious ability to maintain them in conditions which promote their dignity and well-being.

What role should the modern democratic state—on behalf of all its citizens—play in regulating these practices? At present, parents and physicians may be prosecuted when life-saving treatment is withheld. In many instances, the law tends to oversimplify complicated ethical dilemmas. We're not talking about a clear case, like someone swindling pensions away from elderly women. Right and wrong are draped in complex layers of shading; we must delve behind the layers with prudence. It would make more sense to apply moral reasoning on an individual, case-by-case, basis.

An American professor who advocates full state support for the care of severely disabled infants argues that society cannot force parents to preserve the lives of defective newborns against the parents' better judgment. That is, "unless government provides the 'special financial, physical, and psychological resources' necessary to proper treatment of the handicapped child."* I agree with this statement, especially in light of Canada's historical commitment to providing quality and accessible health care for all. My family's experience with publicly funded care has, on the whole, been good but it is also amply evident from our story that, for a variety of reasons, the authorities would prefer to wash their hands of cases once children are sent home from hospital. And that's not good enough.

As Dr. Laura Purdy, a bioethicist at the University of Toronto, said in a recent interview, "I see this as a real moral problem. If we really are going to spend whatever it takes keep certain children alive then (not funding care) does seem hypocritical. If you withdraw support late then what you are really saying is that what matters is biological life. And that the quality of life and happiness and human welfare are actually less important."

We must cast the net of state, i.e. communal, responsibility more widely—beyond the hospital neonatal unit—to include the social and community health services these medically fragile children require during their brief lives. Social policy that provides cradle to grave care, for all children and medically-fragile children in particular, would be a testament to our humanity. Most of these kids have no words. Can we afford to ignore their cries for help?

---

* Joseph Goldstein, quoted in Cantor, *Legal Frontiers of Death and Dying*. See Book List.

13

Who Will Rock My Son?

WHEN I HOLD JAKE I can sit quietly, without defences or armour. He is not squirmy; he cannot jump out of my lap or disobey. The calm I feel with him is akin to what I experience in the woods, which is why I want him to be there, in peace, when his time comes.

Being a parent, whether one's child is ill or healthy, evokes intense feelings of protectiveness. Parenting Jake has meant learning that I cannot defend him—or myself— against his destiny. In that way, he anchors me firmly in the present; it means opening my heart and mind to feel that constant tug, that hurt, but not allowing myself to give in to it. Jake's life has given me a passion to fight for all kids like him. I write articles, organize resistance to social service cuts with other parents and speak out from a position that is profoundly grounded in my experience.

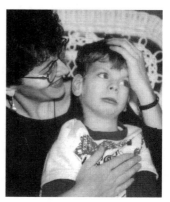

Miriam rocks Jake during a visit to his group home.

It is Jake's vulnerability and his strength, his will to live and, despite all else, his ability to connect deeply with people, that touches us profoundly. Perhaps this is the essence of being human and, in that, he has shared fully and taught us a great deal.

But if you asked me, "Would I wish this on anyone?" the answer would be no. If new research allows people to make a choice when given distressing information during a pregnancy, that choice must be available. But I wouldn't trade Jake for anything. He's the one person in my life who can really keep a secret. Everyone should be so lucky.

A question too rarely asked of parents in our situation is, "What would make it easier for you to parent your son?" The answer is not simple: both ethical principles and practical issues create problems—but they are not insurmountable.

I could only find the care my son needs a two-hour drive from my home. Luckily the highway is good and the winters comparatively short. As well, I am fortunate to have a certain amount of education and a job. English is my first language. I own a car. If I need to stay overnight in Belleville, I can usually afford a motel room. An awful lot of people cannot; many families have longer and more difficult drives. There should be facilities across the country where children like Jake can live close to their families; this is particularly important when a child has siblings. Since his sister's birth, juggling all the competing demands on my (finite) time and energy has proved difficult.

Some families have to wait months, even years, to find a suitable placement for their child. But neither the funding nor facilities are available for many children who should be in complex-care group homes like Jake's. Instead, they are left to lie helpless in hospital beds, often until they die, at four times the cost to the taxpayer.

Hospitals are about illness. They may not provide the individualized programs of infant stimulation or physiotherapy our children require. The hospital's mandate does not include teaching an eight-year-old girl with immense physical and mental challenges to sit on the potty. Well-run group homes, with quality care and consistent staff support linked with medical services, can do this and much more. Coordinated care, delivered through smaller facilities attached to the larger centres of expertise (e.g. medical and psychological services) would benefit many.

Many parents I've spoken with agree that closing down residential care entirely is unrealistic. Some children with disabilities need group home care for at least part of their lives, even if it's only the occasional weekend. Families need opportunities for respite care, for a break from their relentless caregiving schedule, the sort of care available to a few families in Toronto at Thistletown Regional Treatment Centre and the four Safehaven group homes. Why isn't there a network of group homes, easily accessible to parents in all parts of the country? Instead of expanding cost-effective, high quality care, successive governments are cutting back even further on already scarce resources for children with disabilities. In the homes that have been allowed to remain open, budget cutbacks mean resourceful use of funds by administrators like Gail; recently, government regulators did not approve (among other things) the soft mattress pads she lays under the sheets on each of the children's beds to maximize their comfort.

Residential and day programs are in woefully short supply, especially outside of major urban centres. The Metro Agencies Representative Council (MARC) reported waiting lists of thousands in 1995. When I tried to update this information in 1999, I was told that such figures are no longer routinely kept.

MARC also stated in 1995 that one of the largest groups that would be coming through the system was children under five who are "medically complex," those with multiple disabilities who are often dependent on complex equipment to maintain their lives.

Care at Susie's Place costs a quarter as much as hospital care. User fees are now being imposed and the transportation for weekend visits has been discontinued. This is outrageous. These rides— the glue that kept many families together—are being sacrificed to so-called fiscal restraint. And we experience it in isolation, powerless as individuals to protect our kids or integrity as a family. This is, at minimum, benign neglect. At worst, it is nothing short of appalling.

What would a more humane system look like? First, funding would be constant. From the moment it is determined special care is required until death, funding for care should be available without question. It is inhumane to make families jump through hoops every year or, worse, live with great uncertainty while bureaucrats assess and reassess the case at hand. The reassessment process is not only a waste of taxpayers' money, it puts undue strain on families.

Next, children should be able to stay close to their families' homes. People who don't have cars, who can't afford to take time off work, or who have long and—in winter—dangerous drives to make, find it very tough to free up an extra day to make visits. I believe this is an unacceptable burden, causing untold anguish. As well, a child close at hand can be more easily integrated into family activities and can be visited by other family members.

Since a child's (and the family's) needs may change over time, ensuring a network of high quality respite care facilities is crucial for the families of children who are not in full-time residential care. This could be in facilities like Susie's Place in smaller communities or Thistletown in large cities. If parents caring for their severely dis-abled children at home knew they had one week per month as respite, for example, it would be easier for them to sustain their home care schedule. Respite care is a safety valve but not every neighbour or grandparent can pinch hit for parents.

In a humane system, home care would be adequate to families' needs and caregivers would be assigned for longer periods to ease the anxiety families often feel leaving their fragile children with strangers. Continuity of care would also enhance the quality of care as staff would get to know the child and her particular therapeutic and medical needs. The family would benefit from a break and, as a byproduct of coordinated care, would not have to experience the isolation their circumstances often dictate. Reliable services would help families to develop routines, which are particularly hard to maintain in acute care situations.

This means high quality care delivered by trained staff. These dedicated individuals must be compensated appropriately for their professional standards and commitment. If a physiotherapist working for the hospital earns a certain negotiated wage, the same should be paid to the physiotherapist coming into the group home.

Governments' current strategy to privatize home care includes a drive to ratchet down the wages of caregivers in the home. Minimum wage is the goal. Clearly, this is unacceptable. The work is devalued because in many contexts female family members do it for free. Viewing such work as an extension of housework provides a rationale for voluntary, as opposed to paid, labour. Rather, the skilled workers our family members need to survive should be well compensated, just as if they did the same work in an institutional setting.

Achieving this model of care would not be so difficult, if the political will and commitment existed. The cost need not be exorbitant. This kind of facility could be affiliated with a hospital setting in order to access existing resources like occupational and physiotherapy, medical advice, and counselling services. When one child requires so much more attention than others, everyone in the family is affected and it would be useful for siblings to have access to peer support. This is already available to a few families at Thistletown and Safehaven; Bereaved Families of Ontario and its chapters also run groups for children, as well as adults. Parents and entire families may benefit from these services, since the stresses they cope with are both unusual and unrelenting, and in a just society they would be available to Canadians no matter where they live.

This model of care would be based on a "hub," a group home that would function as the access point for families and would be affiliated to a hospital or comprehensive health resource centre.

A related service would be the provision of palliative care for children with severe, life-threatening disabling conditions. Some of these children are kept alive at birth by technology, only to face brief, difficult lives. They need places other than hospitals to live, with dignity, until they die, just as older dying patients may live in hospices.

The group home where Jake resides provides palliative care. One of my first telephone conversations with Gail was to explore how she felt about allowing Jake to die when his time comes. Would she and her staff do everything possible to keep our baby comfortable? Would she ensure that, no matter what, he would never again be anchored to a resuscitator or have a tracheotomy tube pierce his throat?

Gail is experienced in this difficult drill. She offers families the information and support they need to make informed choices about their loved one's care. Doctors from the Children's Aid Society assist. They helped us to understand what was meant by various medical procedures that might be proposed for our son.

This is not mercy killing, to which Gail is absolutely opposed. Nor is the group home a warehouse for society's refuse. Not all of the children die there; some go back to their families, are adopted or move on to foster care. Staff members have even fostered or adopted children to whom they became particularly attached. Other children benefit from competent and loving care until they die at the group home, often in the arms of their caregivers.

Ethical debate and public policy have not yet caught up to the clinical reality that, as medical technology keeps more infants alive, some unfortunate young ones face grim lives. I have described in earlier chapters how doctors at the children's hospital were not willing to enter into dialogue about the possibility of a peaceful or gentle death for our son. Parents must be given full and accurate information about their children's conditions. It means talking through the practical and ethical ramifications of treatments. And it must mean that parents are intimately involved in all levels of their child's care, including the inevitable wrestling with tough decisions.

In Holland, for example, this kind of discussion is encouraged in hospitals among terminally ill patients, their families, and doctors although the outcomes—that is, the percentage of children for whom heroic lifesaving methods are used—are not that different from here in Canada.

The responsibility inherent in doctors' "duty of care" must extend beyond the walls of the institution to include humane care throughout these children's lives—however brief. The "ethic of care" I discuss in the previous chapter provides a sound basis for this shift to more comprehensive social and health policy. The responsibility of the entire community to share with parents the care for medically-fragile children must be fully mandated in legislation; this responsibility to care, of course, would not mean excluding parents from decisions on children's welfare but, rather, providing the family supports appropriate to each particular set of circumstances.

To achieve even a small measure of improvement means families in a range of different situations must come together—as the Thistletown parents did—to establish a political constituency. Together, we must defend our children's needs and protest cuts that compromise our children's care. Governments must not be allowed to use criticisms of how institutions have operated in the past to justify slashing services to the weakest and most vulnerable.

To ensure that social policy catches up with genuine need, people who work in this sector must be involved through their unions and professional associations, along with the families they serve. It is only by creating this kind of political constituency—a voice for our children—that their cries for attention will be heard.

Jake is seriously ill again in January 1998 and as usual I rush to Belleville to be near him. He is on an incredible, awful journey for thirty-six hours, struggling to breathe, to conquer his fever, fighting for his life. As I hold him across my lap, I desperately want him to live while I also want him to be at peace, to be able to die gently, in his own time. When I take a break, the women who have loved and cared for him so long, Cheryl and Gail, hunch over on either side of my boy. He is lying on the floor face down, supported by pillows and wedges, while they give him vigorous chest therapy and suctioning. With their voices, they encourage him to move about and cough. Using a small piece of sheepskin to cushion their touch, they tap his chest and back, jiggling his body. Gail suctions him deeply, through his nose and back into his lungs. Gradually Jake is able to clear some of the mucus backlog and slowly his colour returns to a more normal hue.

By the second evening, he seems to be more peaceful. The fever is breaking, and while I change him, lightly washing him with a damp cloth, he looks up at me with a big smile. All of a sudden, he is back. He has pulled through once again.

Back at work not long after this, I am called to Thunder Bay to meet with a union local at the Lakehead Association for Community Living. I meet many staff and their clients in group homes and day programs of various descriptions. One visit, in particular, touches me deeply.

My guide for the day is Patty, a union member; she takes me through a narrow hallway off the kitchen of the group home where she works to a den. Two women are sitting on a sofa in silence.

The woman nearest to the doorway is close to forty years old, I'd guess. She has dark hair that falls limply to her shoulders. Wearing a navy blue sweat suit, white socks and no shoes, she sits crouched in the fetal position, rocking back and forth on the couch. She does not look up when we enter the room. There is no pause in her rocking. When Patty sits next to her, however, and puts her hands out, the woman shifts into her lap.

Patty rocks her, speaking to me softly. "My supervisor told me not to hold her," she says.

"Why?" I ask. I am curious and, to be honest, I am also upset by the sight of these two women. The second is looking out the window and does not budge from her pose, even at the sound of our voices. Just then, the woman in Patty's lap begins to make deep, guttural sounds. Not words.

"My supervisor does not want us to become involved with the clients," Patty tells me.

I nod.

"But she needs human contact, the same as our kids, don't you think?" Patty says.

As I watch this drama unfold in front of me, my stomach turns somersaults. I'm not proud of my reaction, but nothing has prepared me for this—except perhaps for watching the loving care women like Patty give my son. She goes on rocking this utterly powerless woman most of us would find pathetic, even ugly.

I am horrified by my ability to be so small-minded.

Tonight we will strategize ways for the union local to work with clients and their families to oppose the government's move to close down the group homes and other agency services. Once again, it seems clients will be sent "out into the community" where they can live independently. The union local asks the key question, "Are the necessary supports in place?"

As at Thistletown, committed families who know they are unable to care for their loved ones will meet with the union members concerned. They want to discuss the best approach for ensuring clients continue to receive the care they require, given changing circumstances.

After the meeting, my thoughts drift closer to home. Who will hug Jake if he lives longer than anyone expects? What if Gail has to close down her group home? Would there always be someone as loving as Patty to care for him? To hold him, even if it goes against some policy?

As my son grows older, I realize the gift intrinsic in Gail's care and her promise that Jake may stay for life at Susie's Place. You can't help but feel compassionate toward the sweet babies who come to Gail at a young age but bonding to a big man of a child—should he have to move—is a totally different kettle of fish. Changing the diaper of a thirty-eight-year-old woman is likely a tad unpleasant, at the best of times. I cannot get the thought out of my head, "Who would hold my Jake? Who?"

Every person has the right to receive affection along with basic hygiene and medical attention. It is part of the care these workers provide. They are front-line workers, and often become attached to the people with whom they work. Their needs as workers coincide with the needs of the people they care for.

Is it the union's job to be involved in advocating for the dignity of these more vulnerable people, to ensure that clients receive personal care that includes tenderness or a hug, especially in frenzied times of fiscal restraint?

Unions come out of a tradition of social justice, justice for workers and for the people they serve. In the past, "bread and butter" unionism hasn't included hugs for a severely-challenged woman who rocks back and forth from morning till night. But the professional expertise, as well as the devotion, many trade unionists practice daily makes me wonder whether we should try to negotiate standards of care as well as wage rates.

The qualities that motivate the extraordinary individuals I have had the privilege of working with go well beyond bread and butter. Some are motivated by a spiritual concern, nurtured through their involvement with a particular congregation or set of values. A concern for social justice reflects a recognition of basic rights for all, including those most vulnerable among us; this is inseparable from a belief in the dignity of the human soul—whatever the outward appearance or speech of the person.

Patty told me that the woman she rocked that day has no family. She has no other place to go. How many more people in similar straits are living among us? Do we really want our governments, acting on our behalf, to refuse them decent standards of care?

A few children at Jake's are growing up, their bodies following a predestined path, although other capacities remain limited. One young girl is menstruating. These are children growing like any others. They too need care, love and protection. They cannot speak, but they are crying for our help. It is a sad community moral standard indeed that permits us to ignore them.

In researching the details of Jake's birth, I realised that his father and I had had profoundly different understandings of our son's situation at the time. Jim believed that Jake had been born dead and was then resuscitated.

I was shocked, horrified by this notion. I felt I had been living a lie. All of a sudden, I had a glimpse of Jake as my shadow child, as if I had given birth to a dead bird. I felt soiled, unclean. How could medical science have brought back to life my sweet boy, so fundamentally flawed at birth? How dare they punish him—and us—when he had already found peace. Had I been in love with a person snatched from death's jaws by errant technology?

Today, my Jake is truly gorgeous—and yes, so limited. I cannot assign blame for his condition. He just is who he is—and demands my love.

When I went back to Jake's hospital records, I saw that he was indeed alive at birth. Struggling, but full of life. I felt such relief to learn that I've not been having a love affair with a ghost. This knowledge cleansed my soul, like the cool rain that marks the close of a humid afternoon.

14

Climbing the Stress Meter

OUTRAGEOUS HOUSING COSTS continued to dog us during the early nineties. Here we were, in our prime earning years with children to raise but, even with relatively good incomes, we could scarcely cover basic expenses. No doubt, we were better off than many people in the city. We never had to visit a food bank, although certain items became luxuries. But like lots of ordinary working folks in the early nineties, we were caught. Television news daily reported the unprecedented rate of personal bankruptcies in the country. Although the consumer gorge-fest of the eighties had not been part of our lives we still had to pay the price of its aftermath.

I wanted us to be comfortable in the way my parents strove for: a home to raise a family in, enough stability to plan to have another child, family vacations camping, and music or gymnastic lessons for our kids. I recognize these were middle-class expectations, but it's not a crime to want to live secure lives.

Perhaps our difficulties helped me to write more compelling articles about people who were losing their jobs by the thousands—jobs in Ontario manufacturing plants were biting the dust at the same

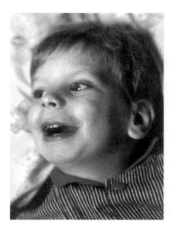

Jake catches the light on a visit home.

time as work in the fishery was disappearing on the East Coast. It is a common myth that the vagaries of the capitalist market build character. But the market also has its victims among working people whose health and family relationships suffer in bad times.

Jim and I were not immune. These pressures put a pall over our otherwise solid partnership. Tension grew. We both found it hard to rekindle the more carefree, hopeful quality of our friendship in early days together.

It is impossible for me to know how much Jake's poor health and guarded prognosis contributed to the distance between us. Certainly Jake—like any child conceived in love—gave us a common sense of purpose. We loved our boy fiercely, engendering a shift in priorities beyond our wildest imaginings. Nonetheless, buying a house together had made us business partners, as well as life mates. This proved much tougher to negotiate, especially since the business was foundering.

In the summer of 1991, I put my foot down. I wanted to leave the duplex on the west side of the city; it was inhabited by a sadness beyond ourselves. I wanted to move closer to Belleville.

Scouring the classified ads for rental properties early each morning, starting before six, became an obsession. I eventually came upon a house with living space for two children in a pleasant community east of downtown and near Lake Ontario, in a neighbourhood called The Beach. The owners of the property were leaving Toronto on a trial basis and wanted someone to care for their home in the interim. We were perfect candidates for this temporary situation.

Moving day arrived just before Jake's first frightening brush with death in the summer after his first birthday. Shortly thereafter, Emma was conceived. Making a fresh start was a powerful impetus. I was thirty-four, Jim was thirty-nine. There was not much respite from the ticking of my powerful biological clock, especially given our bad luck the first time around.

I have already told much of the story of our three years in that house. Economic times in the early nineties were not very favourable to the expansion of progressive social legislation. Life was hectic and full of challenges, both professional and personal. All the same, apart from the finances, these were good times, the first time in many years I had lived in one place for more than a couple of years. I liked feeling settled. The woman at the corner store where we bought milk always asked about the baby. The dry cleaner gave Emma lollipops while we talked fabrics and fashion. I liked the familiarity and friendliness of The Beach. The house was pleasant for entertaining friends and we frequently gathered for a potluck meal or picnic by the lake. We were finally establishing a home base, as if we might plant roots in this community and raise our family here.

When the CBC aired the second radio documentary about Jake on *As It Happens* one early summer evening in 1994, a few neighbours heard it and made the connection to us. It was heartening to be able to share our story with people on the street.

Our babysitter was another link with the neighbourhood. We first met her when Emma was just three months old. Later, she came into the house daily for six months until Emma started daycare. During that time, Emma visited the schoolyard every morning with her sitter whose seven-year-old daughter was in grade two. This helped Emma feel comfortable at the local school; for her, it was like having an older sister, a feeling of connection that has continued to this day. Emma would attend daycare in that school and, once she was old enough, start junior and senior kindergarten in the same building, benefitting from a seamless day. Not having to cobble together alternative care for her during our workday lifted a huge weight off my mind.

I often rode my ancient three-speed blue Schwinn bicycle with Emma's baby seat fastened securely on the back. The bike, which had been mine as a girl in New York, somehow survived the move to Canada, not to mention the ensuing years abandoned in my parent's garage in favor of trim and trendy ten-speed racing models. The Schwinn was perfect for taking Emma for a spin; she loved the feeling of wind on her face and often fell asleep as I pedaled along by the lake.

On winter mornings when it was Jim's turn to sleep in, I would pull Emma in a small pale blue toboggan along the quiet side streets. There was silence except for the scraping of molded hard plastic on snow. Emma would squeal with delight (and sometimes the opposite) as we made our way in the crisp air. I loved those moments walking through our community, listening to the sounds of The Beach awakening.

A sense of rootedness had never been so important to me before. My age was likely a factor; I was tired of drifting like a tumbleweed. In addition to many positive elements, a certain volatility had characterized the emotional landscape of my childhood home. I wanted something different for my own children. Choosing Jim—an exceptionally steady person—as their father, was no accident.

Unfortunately, in the spring of 1994 our landlords put the house up for sale. We knew we would have to move one day but the news was still jarring. One hopes most for stability, especially when circumstances impose the exact opposite. Again, I began my six o'clock morning vigil with the classified pages, scouring both newspapers.

Realtors and prospective buyers began arriving, "trying on" our home. House browsing is a favourite pastime in The Beach. Welcoming gawking tourists into our home disrupted the sense of refuge we had so carefully nurtured. Being civil toward the strangers in our home proved a challenge, especially when Emma's irregular (but oh so precious) nap time was interrupted. When Jake was home, it spelled double trouble. I felt invaded; crankiness is not the sole property of the pre-school set.

Meanwhile, my own house search was proving fruitless, despite early morning phone calls. I could find nothing in The Beach at a rent we could afford. One morning I noticed an ad for a home well to the east of us along the lake, in Scarborough, not far from where my Canadian grandparents had lived until the mid-sixties.

As children, we made the pilgrimage to Toronto two or three times a year, the family packed into the car for marathon driving sessions from New York. We usually crossed over at Niagara Falls or the Peace Bridge, arriving at about seven in the evening, just in time to be greeted and shushed into makeshift cots in my grandfather's study to sleep among his lawyering books and dark mahogany desks.

The owners of the advertised house, on the cliffs high above Lake Ontario, were planning to relocate to the United States. We signed a lease, knowing once more our stay would be short term.

Two house moves in the space of three years demanded lots of energy. I had also just switched jobs, turning up the pressure. While we were not quite a lean, mean fighting machine, Jim and I had got the rhythm of moving down to an art. Our strength was our ability (most of the time) to work as a team; the division of labour around mundane tasks made progress possible. Still, there's no doubt the stress meter was working overtime.

By this time, Emma was scaling stairways and quickly staked out her play area in the basement and backyard. We transferred the entire babyproofing operation to our new abode, complete with portable gates and cupboard locks. Emma soon beat a path from her bedroom to her sleeping father, jumping on him first thing every morning. He was her anchor.

She continued at the same daycare in The Beach and we drove her in each day via a somewhat circuitous route to work. Knowing the next move couldn't be far off, I still hoped to find something back in The Beach community that we could afford to rent.

I sometimes wonder how much the exhaustion from six years of public and private battles for our child's care contributed to the undoing of our marriage. I threw myself into advocating for Jake and children like him. It seemed the least I could do. But it also meant a considerable amount of solitary time writing and pitching my commentaries to newspapers and CBC radio. Jim was often my first and most insightful critic.

But our life as a couple was slowly losing ground to the war room against injustice that had set up camp in the basement study. We were also beginning to look outside our relationship for sustenance and adult companionship: the Jewish women's group and serious writing for me; baseball and running marathons for Jim. These were activities free of the sadness and tension that had come to define our lives together.

Studies show that close to 80 percent of marriages split up after a child has died and, surely, when a child is medically fragile similar stresses are present. Ann Finkbeiner (see Book List) found that couples who divorced grieved separately, each handling loss in their own way: "Bereaved fathers," she says, "put their grief into a compartment separate from the rest of their lives. They feel the need to console and protect their families and so need to submerge their own grief." The distancing I experienced from Jim perhaps reflected our need to find our own ways to recapture a lost innocence. I know he loved our son deeply but suspect that his gender training did not permit him to express it. Years later, he told me that when he walked with newborn Jake through the tunnel from my maternity ward to the Hospital for Sick Children, he felt bereft because he did not know how to protect his raspy little son. I wish he had been able to share those feelings with me at the time; it saddens me still that silence came to divide us like an ocean.

We separated in May 1996. The Scarborough house was up for sale and neither of us could face setting up another home together. The decision to live apart was the culmination of much soul searching. I suspect Jim needed his own space as much as I did. We had grown apart during our ten years together and needed to find a different basis for our relationship. All the same, our respect for one another endured.

But I was tired of my solo assignment on the worry beat, as though I had to shoulder the full burden of concern for Jake by myself. I know Jim did not mean this to happen but ultimately I resented his distance. I was angry; I felt he enjoyed the privilege of hitching his wagon pleasurably to the future—Emma—while I was left behind with our son. And while Jim's reserved nature was terrific in a crisis, I also felt belittled by him for being more expressive.

It is only with the luxury of hindsight that these insights become clear.

In true organizer's fashion I found Jim an apartment several blocks away from the bungalow I moved into with Emma. He and our friends helped to paint and repair my house to a habitable standard. We constructed a clubhouse with swings in the backyard for Emma and her buddies.

Setting up my own home was initially quite liberating. I put posters on the wall that proclaimed, "I am a woman giving birth to myself" and "The soul would have no rainbow if the eyes had no tears." Of course, the initial sense of euphoria and freedom gave way to the mind-numbing exhaustion of life as a single parent. The best advice I received in the early days of our separation was that I would not know what I truly wanted until a significant period of time passed.

Emma lived with me full time at the beginning, seeing her father several times a week. She missed him a great deal and could not understand why we weren't together. I learned to look for practical supports in caring for her and visiting Jake. Once Jim and I developed a routine for sharing time with Emma and were able to disentangle emotionally and financially, the rhythm of co-parenting worked. She now spends a few days a week and alternate weekends at each house. As she gets older we may move to a weekly schedule to allow greater continuity for her with each parent. Our homes are near one another, close to her public school and daycare. There is no question that the consistency in her daily routines helped Emma to move through this difficult transition. Her life outside our homes did not change much as she had a solid group of friends, her babysitter, and teachers who continued to care about her.

Still, my baby girl was just four years old when her father and I split. Blowing her life apart broke my heart. One day, I heard her tell her best friend, "I don't live together anymore." I wanted to cry. She was repeating our words, giving them her own spin.

I tried to help her make the transition, then and now, using colouring books and children's stories about kids with two homes.

She has a calendar in each house that has stickers she attaches to show her schedule so she knows which parent is taking her to swimming or gymnastics that week. Jim and I try to set similar rules about bedtime, allowance and homework. Emma has learned that discipline follows her from one house to the other since Jim and I brief each other on high and low points on the behaviour scale and we hold family meetings when something major must be discussed.

At one point, Emma's highly developed morning dilly-dallying skills became the subject of one such family meeting. Once she came out of hiding in the laundry hamper, we sat together and brainstormed a page of ideas to help her get out of the house more quickly in the morning. She had several ideas and seemed to be taking responsibility for her behaviour. We each signed the bottom of the page and Jim made a copy for each of us. As I left that night, he and I cracked up laughing, realizing we had just signed our first tentative agreement with a five-year-old.

Caring for our son was always a stressful proposition. His life added an unusual dimension to our relationship but the strains we experienced—demanding jobs, cruddy economic times—are things we shared with a large segment of the population. I do not think Jake's condition alone was our undoing. But now, in our changed circumstances, each of our children needs us to maintain a workable partnership; it is the only way we can help them continue to grow into the fine young people they are already becoming.

That first summer on my own was eventful in other ways. The union I work for issued layoff notices to fifty-one staff members, including me. Not only did I have a whopping rent increase in our new digs but I was about to be unemployed. We were forced out on strike. We spent four weeks on the picket line, what Emma called "Mom's picnic line," our children joining us outside the union office in sweltering heat. Colleagues painted the children's faces, adding to the carnival atmosphere. At the end of the job action, we took a significant cut in pay and pension benefits in return for cancellation of the layoffs. It was an appalling situation that should have been avoided.

My friend Frank, who at various times since 1994 has been my boss, has a boy of his own, just a year older than my son. Frank noticed, one winter and spring, that I tended to get particularly antsy every couple of weeks if I hadn't made the trek to Belleville. It was an astute observation, something I knew inside but could not have articulated. What a marvelous gift—especially since he could actually say, "Go, get out of here. That article can wait until tomorrow!"

In our work in the movement we are often convinced that everything we do is vitally important. If there isn't a crisis, we're not doing our jobs. Of course, there's a kernel of truth underlying this mindless propulsion toward activity; unions are, after all, highly political and defensive organizations and, certainly, working people have been under attack. But unfortunately, this drive can also sideline sensible approaches to managing human resources. I've pushed hard during my working life for employers and unions to accommodate workers' family responsibilities. My present employer, OPSEU, is typically quite humane in its approach. This has not always been my experience in the labour movement or elsewhere.

Organizations should structure work so that people with special needs—their families' or their own—can make a full contribution, in a way that is appropriate for them. My own situation has evolved from just family responsibilities to a point where my own health is occasionally in jeopardy. I do what I can to take care of myself and have learned, especially outside the safe harbour of a marriage, that I must rely on a few individuals for mutual support. Practical assistance like driving to Belleville, or the occasional meal together with our kids, goes a long way. But organizations also have to make room for individual solutions without patronizing workers or causing them to feel their livelihoods are at risk.

Often, people with a variety of challenges can do the work just as well with flexible scheduling or with special equipment at their disposal. For those with hidden disabilities such as diabetes, epilepsy or mental health issues, this can be tricky since the symptoms often appear as difficulty coping with job stress. If the work were organized differently, however, such symptoms might not be present.

For example, after my first bout with clinical depression in 1986, I had to relearn some things. My confidence was at a low ebb. Anxiety can block the brain from organizing or coordinating usually mundane tasks, like making a grocery list or following the steps in a recipe. My hands would shake when I took money out of my wallet at the store. My fine motor skills were gone and I felt terribly self-conscious.

Nor could I abide loud noise or crowds. Too much stimulation scared me. I might feel suddenly panicky in a crowded shopping mall or on a busy street. For an organizer and adult educator, this was a huge loss. I was used to going anywhere, addressing groups and classes.

The scariest thing—by far—was not being able to write. I could no longer seem to string together coherent thoughts. I was terrified. I'm no genius, but who was going to hire a middle-aged woman who could neither read nor write? What if my logical mind never came back?

One day my friend Ruth, already quite computer literate in 1986, brought her laptop over and encouraged me to try it. I knew how to type, but I was skeptical. Besides, I was still spooked by the technology.

Gradually, it turned out that with the keyboard, I could write and clear my mind of the rapid thoughts zinging around my brain. Typing out whatever came into my head helped me to express confusing thoughts and feelings. I found I could "empty out" my brain and then make sense of what I'd written.

In my case, a new tool meant that I could manage my work situation even through a stressful period; many people could be helped in a comparable way if their employers were willing to look with them for solutions.

In a related vein, I sometimes feel agitated, as though I were perking away on a caffeine high. Concentrating on reading an article or completing a task can be difficult. At these times, I cover part of the page I am reading with a sheet of plain white paper. This helps me, just as it did when I first learned to read in grade school, to keep my eyes focussed on one line at a time. It doesn't take away the jumpiness

I feel, but this simple reading strategy helps me remain productive.

More recently, I have found, through trial and error, an arsenal of activities that help me to keep my balance in stressful times. Seeing my kids and feeling connected to them is paramount. Taking time for exercise and therapeutic massage is also a requirement.

During the winter, when there is not much light in the day, I wake up at six o'clock and spend time under a full spectrum light, reading the newspaper, before I exercise. At night, I have to start winding down at about nine o'clock during the darkest months. Late meetings or post-meeting debriefs are to be avoided, if at all possible. I no longer drive long distances home from meetings out of town at night. These measures keep me well—although they take time and can be boring as hell. They are limits I have imposed because I must. They help me to manage my own (flawed) constitution.

I know now that it is my responsibility to take care of myself. The song says, "The union makes you strong," and it's true. Working with people to develop collective strategies for change is very important. But the first step is personal responsibility. And the structure of work must be flexible enough to accommodate differences between people, no matter how they manifest themselves.

Our needs as individuals are different but it is nature, and not just our will, that sets the limits on what our bodies can bear. Just as my life is, in fact, enriched by the experience of illness, so too may our organizations be strengthened by taking the reality of human frailty into account. Health and beauty can be fleeting and all working people, including those with disabilities, have the right to reach for the best they can grasp. We must insist, together, that our employers embrace this truth and act accordingly.

15

Balance and Surrender

THE FACT THAT JAKE lives far from home has a tremendous impact on how I approach my life. I miss him constantly; my body aches to hold him. I never know if a visit will be the last.

I am grateful that Jake was my first baby; I didn't know any better than to bond to him fully those months we lived together. That bonding might be harder to achieve with a second or third child. Who would have the time or energy? In a sense, our ignorance provided us a wonderful opportunity to know and love our son. And now, instead of dying, he lives on. One night, a nightmare woke me. Jake was in a baby carriage all alone. I could hear him crying. "Mommy, I need you," I heard him say. I ran but could not reach him in time. He died before my outstretched hand could touch his forehead; he dissolved like a piece of melting toffee and I could not retrieve him.

As I write this, Jake has not died but he has come close many times. Although I am most concerned that he not experience any pain, there is great comfort in knowing that he is cared for by people who love him. The women at Susie's Place are intimately involved in our story. I have wondered, holding Jake all those hours, how I

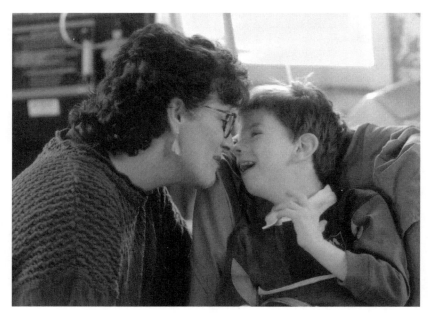

Miriam and Jake share a giggle in Belleville, 1996.

would feel if I were all by myself at home with this fancy equipment around me with only a home care person now and then, a different one each time. I think I would be scared as hell. Instead, I am supported in an otherworldly calm. I can just be with my boy and give him my total attention. I do not have to worry about doing anything wrong, of misreading the machine that monitors his oxygen levels, or even making lunch.

My relationship with Gail is a bit like sharing custody. Even though we come from very different backgrounds—I am a Jew and have been a social activist all my life; Gail's care and love for these kids is informed by her Christian faith—we manage to work with Jake and each other in a way that is respectful. My son and I have gained a caring mother figure; we both benefit from Gail's wisdom and empathy.

It is amazing that Jake is still alive. I am absolutely convinced that his survival is due to the fine care he receives at Susie's Place. He receives comfort care; if he can't stop coughing, he is placed head down with his body draped over a foam wedge. To soothe his cough, his caregivers will place a very small amount of cough syrup on the end of a glycerin stick and swab the back of his throat. If his body is hot from fever, cool baths or sponge baths are given; if he is consti-pated and cranky as a result, he receives a gentle bowel massage. Gail has taught me these procedures so I can be fully involved as a mem-ber of the caregiving team. No matter their challenge, day or night each child is kept comfortable with a combination of medical tech-niques and inventive individual attention.

A few years ago, Jake's seizure medications were not working any longer and he seemed increasingly exhausted by the jolts to his body. He was also quite listless and it was unclear whether this was a medi-cation side effect or exhaustion. The leader of the team of lissence-phaly researchers in the United States told us that there was a treatment alternative. Jake could be admitted to hospital for ten days during which he would receive multiple injections. A series of these shots every three to four months allows some children to function almost seizure-free. But the side effects can be quite complex and hospitalization alone might put Jake at risk as he could be exposed to a new set of infections. In addition to the risks and pain, there was no guarantee the injections would work. Most important, however, treating Jake's seizures would not make him well. He suffers from too many other conditions. It seemed to Jim and me that this treatment would constitute an heroic measure; it went beyond the realm of comfort care. We would not take our son down that road.

Because he is so ill, one can never quite escape the knowledge that each visit might be the last. In the midst of this, I have tried to create rituals that allow me to function as if mothering in an ordinary context. Events like the change of season or observance of the Sab-bath become more important, not necessarily in the way of the fore-fathers, but similar in spirit. I find I increasingly need to mark all that is regular or predictable—like the setting of the sun—as a way, per-haps, of handling all that is not, including Jake's health.

Given a choice, I would never live apart from either of my chil-dren. But it is in this circumstance that I must help them grow sturdy roots, so they may flourish.

Blue hydrangeas always remind me of Jake's birth. I recall a feeling of great buoyancy the spring he was born. Each year around his birthday in April, I pick up a pot of blue hydrangeas like the ones Jim's father sent to my hospital room in 1990. Later in the spring, near Mother's Day and Emma's birthday in May, I choose another pot of pink or lavender ones to plant in our garden. We always have hydrangeas at Passover.

Jim was reluctant to participate in these rituals I developed for myself, to mark important dates in the lives of our children. I suspect they seemed overly sentimental to him. For a long time I envied his ability to live in the present, no matter what, and to just keep going.

He is supportive of my wish for Emma to attend a secular humanist Jewish heritage program on Sunday morning, a school much like the one I attended as a child in New York. It stresses secular values, strong ties to cultural traditions and holidays, and encourages respect for diversity. Some of our friends are also part of the *shule* community, including several interfaith and gay and lesbian families.

Most of all, it is wonderful to discover that Emma and I know some of the same songs. One day I heard her singing from the back of the car a Chanukah song in Yiddish I had learned at about the same age. Similarly, at a *shule* family event one day she recognized the tune and Hebrew lyrics from a song I had sung to both her and Jake as babies, while rocking them to sleep.

One Sunday when Emma had been at the *shule*, we got together with my parents and my brother's family to celebrate a birthday. Emma looked across the table at her Grandpa Howard, a man of 82, and said in Yiddish, "Meine nomen es Emma. Vos is deine nomen?" There was a momentary lapse in all conversation. My father quickly recovered from his surprise and answered her while the rest of us cracked up.

It is April 12, 1999. Emma and I are sitting at the community third Passover Seder in Toronto. We are surrounded by other families and friends, most of whom are connected with the *shule* that

Emma attends. The story of Passover is told in songs and poetry. Current events in Canada and beyond, including liberation struggles in Palestine, Yugoslavia and Latin America, are woven into the evening's observance.

As my daughter runs between my lap and the choir at the front of the room when it is her class's turn to sing, I am filled with a sense of well-being. Sitting at the table with us is the new man in my life, along with many of the friends who have been with us for Pesach in other years and for Jake's five-year-old Bar Mitzvah.

Emma revels in stories recounting how she ran all over this dining hall as a toddler, climbing up to join the kids singing, even though she barely knew the songs. She takes a friend over to meet her *shule* teacher. Emma is the big kid this year, and insists on having the grown-up Hagaddah, the book which tells the story of Passover, rather than the colouring book version that features puzzle pages and connect-the-dot exercises.

She has already asked my parents to attend this Seder next year so they may hear her sing. She would also like her Dad to come again to the Seder with us.

"How come Daddy and Uncle Mark aren't here?" she asks me.

"Not this year," I say. "But maybe another year they can join us."

Emma says okay, accepting the line I've drawn. I think about our reconstituted family a lot and I want so badly for the Seder to be a special memory for her. But I don't want it marred for me this year by the ghost of failed relationships. Maybe next year I'll be ready to set our family blender at high speed!

This is the first year I've come with a date; my friend knows a number of the activists there. I feel comfortable; maybe I am ready for yet another transition.

It is a very public event. Usually I feel quite churned up by meeting the large numbers of people here while I marvel at the curious ways in which our lives intersect. Tonight, however, everything feels fine. As I listen to the young tenor who belts out songs in Yiddish, I feel soothed and fundamentally rooted in this expressive urban community.

I want Emma to enjoy this feeling of community too. Tonight she is in her element, running around with the kids and playing. And since she is old enough not to tumble head-first down the stairs, I don't have to keep an eye on her every second.

In the middle of the Passover story is a passage where the ten plagues are recited. These include darkness and the slaying of the first-born. My heart is suddenly struck by a pang of longing for Jake. I wish he were closer, sitting with us at this Seder table. Of course, he isn't. I suddenly recall my first introduction to the community Passover in April, 1990, when he was kicking up a storm in my big round belly. He was due only a couple of weeks later.

Tonight I notice the number of times this Seder refers to building a better world. This is the very message that permeated the dinner table in my parent's home, the message that propelled me into my chosen field as a union representative. I realize that it is, in fact, the telling and retelling of the Passover story that informs my own commitment to making the world a better place. I am still very attached to that message and yet I hope that my daughter will feel freer to choose than I did. Serving others, unless you have a very clear sense of your own psychological boundaries and capacities, can be both enervating and destructive of self. I know that territory. More than once I have felt burnt out by the work, perhaps because I did not know how to build enough nurturing into my life. Feeling a sense of community around me as I do here, counts for something. That is why I seek it much more deliberately now.

Several days later, I awake feeling troubled. My sleep is fitful, again. Outside my window, the jewelled beginning of the day unfolds. A squirrel is scampering across the tattered garage roof set just behind our house. Why do I feel so uneasy? Have those damned raccoons ransacked the garbage cans again?

I shift my gaze to the bookshelf near the bed. My watch says April 22, 1999. I quickly take mental stock. The house is still. I can't hear Emma's faint snoring from her room next to mine. Of course, she's with her father this weekend. Jake is with Gail in Belleville. There have been no phone calls so everyone must be all right.

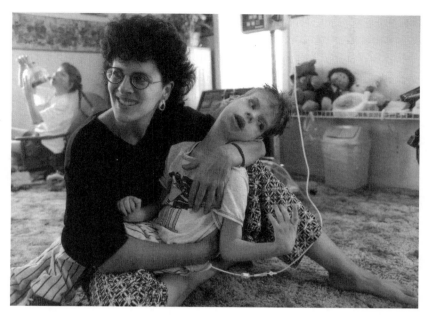

Miriam and Jake have a cuddle in the playroom, 1996.

Suddenly, I recall last night's dream, vivid and disturbing.

In tears, I had implored my son, "Jake, please. Release me."

My voice is cracking, veiled in sadness but with an unfamiliar hard edge.

"Please, Jakey. I can't go on like this."

Fully awake now, I sit straight up in bed. I feel only shame. How selfish! What kind of mother must I be?

And then my son's dream words come to me.

"Mommy, it's okay," he says sweetly. "You can be happy, I want you to."

Stunned, I lie back down and cover my head with a pillow. How could I have said that to my son? *Release me?* Sounds like a bad version of a Bob Dylan song.

That evening, as the embers in the fireplace pierce the blanket of night, I'm aware of a new sensation. Something is opening inside of me, a new possibility.

Can it be that Jake is so wise? It's true that his father and I were unable to cradle the sadness of our lives in our hands. Even the joy we shared raising Emma couldn't bring back the innocence we had lost somewhere along the way.

I know now in ways I never before understood that Jim turned away from our marriage and my sense of us as a family long before I was ready. I thought we would say goodbye and move on. The abyss of darkness I encountered some months after our split proved an unwelcome surprise.

I had underestimated what it meant to lose my partner's support in raising our little girl. But it is only now, three years and many tears later that my anger begins to dissipate. It finally sinks in that I too can turn the page without losing myself, or Jake and Emma. My children will always be with me, each in their own way. Just as they carry me within their hearts.

"Are you ready to let your son go?" someone asked me recently. To be honest, I doubt if I'll ever be ready to let him go. But if it's his time, I will have to accept it. No doctor can fix Jake. When it's time, he has to be free to go gently. Just as he came into the world when it was time, he has to be allowed to go out, serenely, I hope.

I have had to face the nearness of his death many times. My usual coping mechanism for these crises is to be an organizer. I spend a lot of time working out how to care for Jake in his last days, and after he dies. Caring for him has included planning a memorial service. After the lissencephaly researchers have an opportunity to examine his brain, Jake will be cremated.

Close friends will take part in the service, lead the ceremony, helping with flowers and other arrangements; Leo will say a few words about the meaning of Jake's life. Making these plans is part of creating community; doing it alone would be much sadder. The memorial service will give us all a chance to say goodbye. What is said about his short life and our struggles as a family will celebrate Jake and all he has given us.

Jake continues to tie Jim and me together. Even as we were preparing to set up separate households a few blocks apart, we met the rabbi at a synagogue downtown to plan Jake's service. The synagogue is quite small and modestly lined with pine. It felt right to share this painful process with Jim, right through to the end. We decided to ask the rabbi to say a traditional prayer about Jake's soul and to sing the Kaddish, the Jewish prayer for the dead. I want to hear the cantor sing; I wish to be enveloped in that sacred music that lends a brief space for mourning filled with beautiful sounds, not words.

Jim and I agreed that we will invite our friends to gather to sit shiva after our son's death, to honour him and rejoice in his life. As it says in the Song of Songs, "Why should (we) wander in sadness among the herds of (our) friends?"

After our son is cremated, Jim and I will scatter his ashes on the lake in the Gatineau Hills. Jake was there when I was six months pregnant and Jim and I showshoed across that lake. We also spent a couple of days there when he was a tiny infant, before we received his diagnosis. Jakey has always responded to the sound of birds singing and when the loons call I will know he is there. Although I never before thought this way, I imagine now that after his death, Jake's spirit will be free, merging with the pure northern waters, just as he was safe and whole in the waters of my womb, where he could breathe without struggle. He will at last be free to wander, in peace.

Reason tells me that there will be some relief for me when he dies but I'm not ready in my heart to accept that finality. Certainly I will be less tired because I won't be running back and forth, but I will miss him. I will miss the calm that comes to me while holding my son. His coos bring me a sense of peace; the problems of the world melt away. All that exists with Jake is the moment itself. And I will certainly miss the clarity of purpose he has given my life during these years together.

In my need for ritual, I am thinking about carrying out the Orthodox Jewish tradition whereby mourners say the Kaddish prayer every day in synagogue for one year after a loved one's death. I don't have to decide right away. In fact, I am uneasy, searching to identify my own comfort level with certain options. Do I truly want Jake to be cremated? Don't we need a grave site here in Toronto that we can visit? What about the prohibition on cremation observed by religious Jews? I realize that this internal debate is part of my ongoing mothering process; it is how my mind tries to care for my son, by thinking through and analyzing every possibility.

More concretely, I need to find a container for Jake's ashes, something special, solemn but reflecting the generosity of the earth and its elements. When I have had this desire before I haven't acted on it, too overcome by the finality it implies. But last summer, I purposely made a trip to an open-air art fair. The square in front of Toronto's City Hall was full of beautiful objects, paintings, and jewellery. I criss-crossed the aisles, looking for an urn I could cherish.

There were so many choices and colours. Different textures and shapes abounded at every artist's booth. I am usually drawn to simple lines and hues like the earth tones I love. Finally, a small reddish-brown container captured my attention. Would it hold my child's small body? The lid was secure and it had a comforting texture. In my hands, it felt sturdy yet elegant.

This was the one. I brought it home and placed it on the mantle in my living room knowing I have crossed yet another bridge on this journey with Jake.

The knowledge of difficult transitions informs my memories. I recall a day in 1997 when I lay in the grassy hollow behind Susie's Place near where the scraggy conifer forest begins. The hard-packed brown dirt on Baptist Church Road, where Emma took some of her first steps, is only yards away. A line of poplars stands straight as pins. The sky that day was majestic, dark clouds swooping vast distances, a summer storm brewing.

The uneasy weather breeds a certain humility. Not unlike Jake's life, the outcome overhead is beyond human control. I am reminded that spirituality exists in everyday acts, in living simply.

At six years old, Jake lost four baby teeth. Such irony—it's as if no one told his body to quit growing so normally. He resembled any other young boy, lanky and lean, a reminder of how tall he would be if he could stand. His body is following a preordained path, not heeding the warning signs. Clearly the urge to survive burns strongly in the genetic information we each carry.

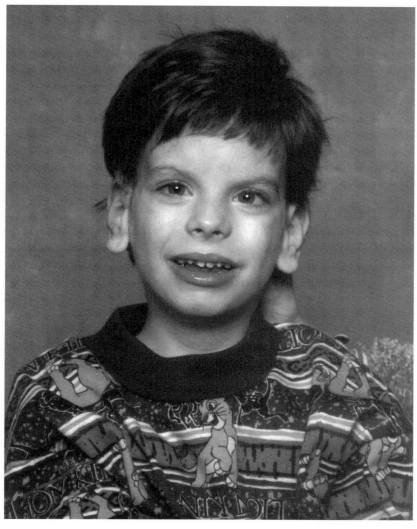

Jake, age 7½ (with a little help from friends!).

Jake was so long, so tall at seven years, his dangly limbs jutting about in untraced movements. Soft hair the colour of rust sprouted on his legs. He was, and always is, dressed attractively in boyish, sporty clothes. While his spirit remains strong, his features are soulful. What has this boy seen in his short life? How would *he* recount his story? I only know that his words would rivet me and that I would listen gratefully, in rapture, for hours on end.

Later the same summer, at the lake in the Gatineau Hills with Emma, the inevitable black flies are the least of my concerns. The annoying bugs eventually depart, leaving a much desired silence. Except this year, the stillness is overwhelming. My marriage is over; the cottage, on the land which I loved years before I knew Jim, is mine. Now I must remake our life here to fit our changed circumstances.

At the cottage again the following summer, Emma and I sit on the flat expanse of rock that layers the shoreline. The waters are still and I am in awe of the serenity this relative wilderness induces. Looking over the trees on the other side of the lake, rose and violet hues mark the horizon where the sun has dropped. I explain to Emma that the pink sky means tomorrow will be a nice day. She smiles, lost in her own sleepy reverie. It's been a long day.

I recognize, gratefully, that my daughter and I have emerged intact. After all the tears (mine) and acting out (both of us), Emma and I are now well and, at times, thriving. It's as if we spent the last year on a swirling amusement park ride. It shook us up and then spat us out, miraculously whole, leaving behind magnificent shattering turbulence. I am proud of my new-found strength and will continue to care for my daughter with all the heart and mind I can muster.

In that moment I am suddenly conscious that it is in the smiles of my children—one brimming with health and one struggling at death's door—that I find the promise of days to come. This is a simple truth, of course. For it is in the brightness of their smiles and depth of their souls that I rest my hopes for the future.

Resources for Parents

Useful Books

For parents and other adults

These are very practical, not theoretical, titles; some of them are mentioned in the text. This list is not exhaustive but you might find it helpful.

Batshaw, Mark L. *Your Child Has a Handicap: A Practical Guide to Daily Care*. Boston, Mass: Little, Brown and Co., 1993.

Clarke, Patricia et al. *To A Different Drumbeat: A Practical Guide to Parenting Children with Special Needs*. Hudson, N.J.: Anthroposophic/Hawthorn Press, 1989.

Diamant, Anita. *Saying Kaddish: How to Comfort the Dying, Bury the Dead & Mourn as a Jew*. New York, NY: Schocken, 1999.

Finkbeiner, Ann K. *After the Death of a Child: Living with Loss Through the Years*. New York, NY: Simon and Schuster, 1996.

Good, Julia P. and Joyce Good Reis. *A Special Kind of Parenting: Meeting the Needs of Handicapped Children*. Schaumberg, Il: La Leche League International, 1985.

Krajicek, Marilyn, et al., eds. *Handbook for the Care of Infants, Toddlers, and Young Children with Disabilities and Chronic Conditions*. Austin, TX: Pro-Ed, 1997.

Kushner, Harold S. *When Bad Things Happen to Good People*. New York, NY: Avon, 1983.

Maurice Lamm. *The Jewish Way in Death and Mourning*. New York, NY: Jonathan David, 1994.

Siegel, Bryna and Silverstein, S.C. *What About Me: Growing Up with a Developmentally Disabled Sibling*. New York, NY: Plenum Insight Books, 1994.

Simons, Robin. *After the Tears: Parents Talk about Raising a Child with a Disability*. San Diego, CA: Harbrace, 1987.

Sweeney, Wilma K. *The Special Needs Reading List: An Annotated Guide to the Best Publications for Parents and Professionals*. Bethesda, MD: Woodbine House, 1998.

For adults and children

Prestine, Joan S. *Someone Special Died* (Picture book and resource guide). Columbia, OH: Fearon Teacher Aids, 1993.

Kroen, William C. *Helping Children Cope with the Loss of a Loved One: A Guide for Grownups*. Minneapolis, MN: Free Spirit Publishing, 1996.

Wolfelf, Alan D. *How I Feel: A Colouring Book for Grieving Children*. Fort Collins, CO: Companion, 1996.

For children

I have always read Emma age-appropriate books about kids with disabilities to help her be aware that lots of children have different challenges. These are some of our favourites:

Brown, Laurene K. and Marc Brown. *When Dinosaurs Die: A Guide to Understanding Death*. Boston, MS: Little, Brown and Co., 1996.

Cairo, Shelley, Jasmine Cairo and Tara Cairo. *Our Brother Has Down's Syndrome: An Introduction for Children*. Toronto: Annick Press Ltd., 1985.

Fleming, Virginia. *Be Good to Eddie Lee*. New York, NY: Putnam, 1993. About a boy with Down's Syndrome.

Osofsky, Audrey. *My Buddy.* New York, NY: Henry Holt and Co., 1992. About a boy with muscular dystrophy. He is in a wheelchair and has a dog as an attendant.

Wright, Betty Ren. *My Sister is Different.* Raintree Steck-Vaughn, 1991. About a girl who is mentally challenged and her brother.

Zelonky, Joy. *I Can't Always Hear You.* Raintree Steck-Vaughn, 1991. About a girl who is hearing impaired.

Books on Bioethics

Cantor, Norman L. *Legal Frontiers of Death and Dying.* Bloomington and Indianapolis: Indiana University Press, 1987.

Dickens, Bernard. "Medicine and the Law—Withholding Pediatric Care." *Canadian Bar Review* 62 (1984).

Gilligan, Carol. *In a Different Voice: Psychological Theory and Women's Development.* Cambridge, MA: Harvard University Press, 1982.

Mullens, Anne. *Timely Deaths: Considering our Last Rights.* Toronto: Knopf Canada, 1996.

Noddings, Nel. *Caring: A Feminine Approach to Ethics and Moral Education.* Berkeley and Los Angeles: University of California Press, 1984.

Ruddick, Sara. *Maternal Thinking: Toward a Politics of Peace.* Boston, MA: Beacon, 1994.

Sherwin, Susan. *No Longer Patient: Feminist Ethics and Health Care.* Philadelphia, PA: Temple University Press, 1992.

Tyson, Jon. "Evidence-Based Ethics and the Care of Premature Infants." *The Future of Children*, vol.5, no. 1 (Spring 1995).

Weir, Robert. *Selective Non-Treatment of Handicapped Newborns: Moral Dilemmas in Neonatal Medicine.* New York, NY: Oxford University Press, 1984.

Wolf, M., ed. *Feminism and Bioethics: Beyond Reproduction.* New York, NY: Oxford University Press, 1996.

Suggestions for Parents

1 Many hospitals have a patient advocate or ombudsperson. Contact this person, even if only as a source of support and for help in dealing with the hospital bureaucracy.

2 There may be a parents' support group in the hospital or in your community. If you don't have a conclusive diagnosis yet, contact a group that deals with a condition similar to your child's. For example, when my son was having seizures, I found the epilepsy foundation very helpful. Public health nurses or the hospital social workers may have information about such groups.

3 Search out the palliative care nurses at the hospital. They have plenty of good information and are not afraid to discuss the tough issues many doctors tend to avoid.

4 If necessary, make an appointment to see the hospital's bioethicist to discuss your child's situation. You have the right to be given as much information as you need on every procedure planned.

5 Disability organizations exist in many communities. You will find them listed in the phone book or by asking hospital social workers. Public health nurses should also have this information.

6 The Internet is a marvelous information source. Many disability organizations have extensive web sites with lots of practical information and useful contacts.

7 Contact your local women's resource centre; they often have information about active self-help groups in the community. They will often help you to organize support for yourself and your family.

8 Do not be afraid to ask for help. Your minister or rabbi may be of assistance. There may also be a counsellor or therapist in your community with experience in disability issues.

9   The local Children's Aid Society or child treatment facility may also be aware of services that can help your other children to adjust to new family circumstances. In my community, for example, the CAS runs a siblings group.

10 The important thing to remember is that you did nothing wrong. In time you will regain your equilibrium and find peace of mind. In the meantime, reach out. You are not alone and your friends may be able to put you in touch with a network of other families who will have useful knowledge to share.

How to be most helpful to someone who learns their child is severely disabled or may die

1   Offer practical help—even little things count. If the child is in hospital, offer to relieve the parents at his/her bedside. Offer to take the other children into your own home for meals or on outings. Bring a ready-cooked meal to the family's home. Drive the other children to school or sports activities.

2   Help your own children, gently, to understand the other family's special needs. Your example, your comfort level is an important model. Frank discussion and explanations of any strange equipment help to assuage children's fears. Disability organizations, hospital social workers, a children's or parenting bookstore can direct you to age-appropriate books.

3   Encourage the family concerned to express its worries, even if it is painful for you to listen. Your support will be invaluable—sometimes just listening is enough. Other times, it may be helpful for you to offer more practical assistance.

4   Support decisions made by the family. You do not know the depth of their feelings and cannot judge their actions but your support will certainly help them through tough periods.

5 Include the child in community celebrations and birthdays. Select gifts that are appropriate to his/her abilities. My son, for example, often receives brightly-coloured mobiles or cuddly objects, or toys that make music. Encourage your children to make gifts like these for their friend or family member.

Advice to Professionals

1 Listen carefully to the parents and family. They know their child best. Their observations and knowledge of the child's health problems should be an integral part of any treatment plan.

2 Give full explanations of diagnosis, treatment options, and relevant therapies. Explain medical procedures and concerns in detail. Families want truth, above all, about their child's condition. Do not patronize.

3 Do not imagine for a second that you understand what these families are going through. Your role is to facilitate the person's care. This is only possible if you develop a partnership with family members.

4 Have reading lists and other resources available for the family, in English and other languages. These should include explanations written in plain language covering diagnosis and treatment options. Age-appropriate materials for children are particularly important.

5 Be aware of any community resources available to the family. Provide this information early so they may maximize their support circle.

6 Developing a relationship of trust with the family may take some time. Be patient. They may have already bounced around the system and need time to learn to trust your advice.

7 Where possible, put parents in contact with other families that have faced similar situations. These contacts will be invaluable.

8 Remember that humility (yours) is a virtue. It is the parents who will have to shoulder the extraordinary challenges of raising their special needs child. You should seek to empower the parents by sharing relevant information and treating them with respect.